Staying S[illegible]

How to Control the Drink Demon

Binki Laidler

Published by Accent Press Ltd – 2014

ISBN: 9781783754304

Acknowledgements

This book is dedicated to the good folk of soberistas.com. I salute you all with my glass of sparkling water and thank you from the bottom of my sober heart for your input.

Thank you to Lucy Rocca and Sarah Turner who wrote the life changing book The Sober Revolution and created the amazing site Soberistas. All four saved me.

Thank you to professional writer Darren for his fantastic help. Thank you to professional writer Kate, also a dear friend, who encouraged me to write and gently pushed me along.

Thank you to Cat Camacho of Accent Press who made this book what it is and helped me count to 100.

Thank you to my other half (OH), who put up with my moods forever, and always told me I could do this, and had to make his own omelettes while I wrote.

Thank you to Nicki and Linda who reached out to me and make me laugh every single day and who are partly responsible for my sobriety. Thank you to the many other inspirational ladies who give me the time of day like Laura, Kim, Anghared, Expatmum, and Pip, and many more who I wish I had space to mention; all those sisters who look after me and who are incredible, beautiful women and often don't even know it, and whose lovely feet smoothed down the path for me, following on.

Thank you to the doctors, emergency services, addiction agencies, and domestic violence organisations in the UK and elsewhere in the world, doing a terribly difficult job and far too often having to clear up the god-awful mess resulting from drinking alcohol. I hope one day someone who writes the cheques does more to help you. Thank you to me for believing in myself.

Foreword

I have suffered depression and anxiety on and off all my life. When I think of my childhood, I can remember vast swathes of time where I was worried about one thing and another. I was afraid that I didn't fit in at school with anyone, even my friendship group, and likewise at university. I worried about being misrepresented by people who were supposed to have my back. There was anxiety about my capacity for blistering anger. Finally, of course, there was worry that as a young teen and onwards I could not seem to stop drinking.

When I married my first husband, I was always afraid of being beaten and humiliated by him if I stepped out of line, which I always seemed to do. I was worried about him having affairs and lying to me, and of course it was because I was a terrible person and a useless wife. I worried that my pub habit had developed into daily bottles in the house, and no longer just in the evening.

I worried about not being able to focus at work because I was constantly hungover and simply waiting to get home to a drink. I started my working life in PR, where socialising and drinking were almost a requirement of the post. Later, as a teacher, long hours and continuous stress were a breeding ground for bottles of red. Bouts of depression led to too much time off and self-medicating with the old vino increased. I was an accident waiting to happen, and eventually it did. My drinking immediately before horse riding led to a snapped femur and a year off work, to add to all the other sick leave I had taken.

I worried that people didn't like me and consoled myself, alone, with alcohol. I worried about being lonely to my core for the rest of my life and that red wine had somehow become my best friend. Worried that everyone else was having children and doing normal stuff where I remained childless – I couldn't have my children worried like me; that would be too cruel.

It was this constant anxiety that led me to drinking to excess, and it is only in recent months that I have finally got a handle on it, leading me focus on recovery and to record the first hundred days of my sober journey in the pages which follow.

I don't feel worried with my lovely second husband. He is the love of my life. I trust him with everything. He doesn't generate worry in me. Worries are just ordinary stuff, like getting enough shopping in for the weekend and the quickly-mounting housework. I don't worry about coming home to find him gone, or him turning on me out of the blue, playing mind games because he enjoys it. He would never hurt me; I know that with absolute conviction. He likes the fact that I am me, even though I puzzle him. I am lucky, although I had to wait a long time for my soul mate.

It was the website Soberistas, a social network for people who want to give up alcohol, which rescued me, plain and simple. I came across it entirely by accident, using the search 'how to stop drinking', as I suspect many have done before and since. I could never have quit drinking alone, I had tried too many times in the past, and each time I failed, my resolve for the next time weakened a little more. Blogging on Soberistas, receiving feedback, and making new sober friends were all lifesaving developments. With the sense of community on the site, I made it.

At the time of writing, I am forty-seven immature years old and would rate myself in my drinking days as an addict who loved the thought of being pissed but was never any good at it. I was a rubbish drinker but kept practising. I had several hundred attempts to give up before July 19th 2013, when I finally decided enough was enough and I was having my last ever alcoholic drink. This book recounts my diary and blogs during the first one hundred days, and I am happy to report at the time of writing I am still happily AF (alcohol free).

Please be aware that there are some distressing incidents described in this book involving domestic violence and sexual assault, where the Drink Demon, the one who enticed me to over-indulge, was ever present, and you should not read on without being ready to deal with how this might affect you. I have included the worst elements of my drinking years because I want women, particularly younger women, to be in no doubt at all about how dependent drinking puts us in danger, causes us to lose our judgment or any accurate assessment of other people's true character or intentions, and wrecks our mental health for many years after. And it made me fat and wobbly.

Follow Binki's sober life on
sobernoodles.wordpress.com *and on* Soberistas.com

Introduction

I read many messages online from people who say things like: I am not as bad a drinker as my friends/family/colleagues. Or maybe they talk about the term 'alcoholic' and dismiss the word as simply not applicable. They just like a drink, nothing more, but they don't dare test the calm waters of sobriety for more than a couple of days, because deep down they know there are currents they simply won't be able to handle.

I too spent hundreds of years telling myself that my drinking was never as bad as Miss X or Mr Y. I still had my driving licence and didn't have red veins covering my face like a web. I hadn't been to rehab, nor received treatment from my doctor for alcoholism. I didn't fight in the street or vomit in people's gardens. I had been to AA twice but hated it; therefore I wasn't one of them.

Yet I was sinking, slowly but surely. I focused less, worked less, achieved less. I didn't really interact with people any more. Most of my evenings were a woozy blur, asleep by nine, but awake and sore headed at two in the morning. The depression which had followed me around like my personal raincloud seemed to have lodged itself firmly over my head. If I managed a night of two 'off the drink' I felt rather pathetically proud of myself. The fact that the next time I drank, the whole bottle would disappear in a few greedy slurps was conveniently forgotten. I realised that even if others drank more and loved it, making comparisons was self-destructive. After thirty years of excess, I had had enough.

I first decided I had to finally finish this addiction when I had been married to my second husband for about three months, because I had ruined a lovely day and night by too much drink.

This epiphany occurred after me getting pissed in the house and disappearing without a word to him, in the worst snowstorm for twenty years, to meet old drinking buddies for more alcohol, and having to stay at a friend's (read drinking partner's) because no taxis were running in the hideous weather. On my return, shamefaced the next day, he having had no idea where I ended up, we both cried so many tears and I felt so upset, angry, selfish, and so many other emotions. He left the house and said he needed a drive for half an hour to really think and I honestly thought he was going to leave for ever.

I begged and pleaded for another chance and the sadness in his eyes told me I had almost pushed too far. After he'd gone, I went to the kitchen and threw all the empty cans and bottles all over the kitchen floor and it hit me that I had chosen drink over us.

When he finally came back from his alone time, to my great relief he told me he was giving us another chance; he loved me so much but couldn't bear to stand and watch me hurt myself with drink.

This wake-up gave me the strength I needed. But it still took two more years of trying to moderate and putting myself through mental agony of daily fights before I accepted I had to become an alcohol-free zone.

Another factor in this being the final time I gave up alcohol were the many disease symptoms that I suffered after drinking. I had some investigations earlier in the year I quit and was diagnosed with diverticular disease. This is a recurring bowel infection where the bowel has stretched and formed pockets (sorry to be icky). It causes pain and other distressing problems and can lead to a life-threatening rupture of the bowel, or even be a preceding illness to bowel cancer. I noticed it was particularly bad after heavy bouts with the old red wine and then it started to happen after even a small amount of any alcohol, crippling me sometimes and leading to a lot of time getting doctor's notes for work, which did my reputation no good at all. Since I packed in the drink I hadn't had any attacks and most of the time everything functioned regularly.

I get very sad when I read that people are struggling with the thought of drinking and that life is getting too much without a drink to make it all go away. In this book I want to share the thought processes I experienced whenever I suffered the urge to drink. I hope some elements of my writing will encourage others to develop their own thinking (as opposed to drinking) routine.

This is how my thoughts go:

Step 1. I want a drink. For me, a beautiful half pint of red wine in an elegant huge wine glass (my OH calls it a Brian Potter glass from *Phoenix Nights*, the one that was bigger than every other glass in the building).

Step 2. I tell myself it is one glass of wine, it is enough to satisfy and I will not have another one. I just need to have that one to take the edge off the shit that is my life.

Step 3. I go to the corner shop and spend my £5.99 and bring my treasured bottle back to the house, hardly able to wait till I get in the door before I twist off the cap (it's that kind of wine) and cannot pour it quick enough into my Brian Potter glass.

Step 4. I take a well-earned sip and ignoring the back taste and the tannin and the burn at the back of my throat, think 'that is wonderful'. I top up the glass again so that when I sit down with my treasure (cue voice of Gollum and his obsession with the ring) I have a full glass rather than a rather disappointing half full one (it was a big initial sip).

Step 5. The ruby red liquid calls out to me so I find myself taking pretty long gulps, because after all it is one glass I am allowing myself and one glass only, and I need it in me. The telly and the conversation my husband is trying to engage me in really don't matter, as long as I achieve the relief I am seeking with the wine.

Step 6. The glass is empty. I now feel deeply dissatisfied and twitchy. Was that it? Am I not supposed to feel good now? Didn't I tell myself one glass would do the trick? I need a bloody cigarette now to take away the anxiety caused by restricting myself to one (large) glass of my friend. OH sighs and frowns when I go on the back step and have a smoke, walking past that half-full bottle and thinking, it cost me £5.99, so I cannot justify pouring it down the sink.

Step 7. By the end of the tab, I think fuck it, I am going to finish the bottle and that will be it, the thing is done, I will carry on as normal tomorrow. So I take my Brian Potter glass and fill it up a second time.

Step 8. This second glass doesn't feel so pleasurable; it feels more like a spot of desperation. I feel half pissed, tired, wanting another ciggie, argumentative, and need to lie on the sofa and stare at the telly, at a programme I am not even half interested in. I force it down, aware of the minging taste and my body feeling like it has been run over, and then the munchies come and I eat a pile of shit to offset the cravings and feelings of frustration that are coming at me from all directions.

Step 9. Feel like crap, keep dropping off, go to bed, ignore husband who is trying to hold his tongue but his face says it all.

Step 10. Fall unconscious until waking, hoping it is morning, look at my little alarm clock and it is 2 a.m. I feel dizzy, sickly, craving sugary stuff, so thirsty I fear my throat will crack, tongue so swollen it fills almost my entire mouth, whole body aching with the effects of being poisoned. I consider having alcohol to make me drop off again. I lie there for a couple of hours before grabbing a little more sleep and then the alarm goes and I have to get ready for the day.

Step 11. Hangover. Moderate hangover, but still enough to ruin my day. Am ratty with OH, eat fattening shite food, look at myself and see a distended belly, bags under eyes, watery eyes, pale skin, turned-down mouth with the sadness of it all. Snappy and impatient with people, need to be alone, get very little done that I had planned. Clothes feel uncomfortable and wrong, hair won't do as it is told, skin leeches alcohol and sweat all day. Even a hot bath doesn't sort it out.

Step 12. Get through a hellish crappy day in a snappy mood, having to pretend all day I am OK. By 5 p.m. I am again thinking about drinking to take the hangover away. It starts again – one drink will do the trick, make me feel better, take away the pain and shame for a little while. Just one drink. I know I am lying to myself again and I will disappoint my partner again and get nothing done again and wish I was dead again.

Step Lucky 13. I decide to wipe out steps 1-12 and not even go there. And the relief of knowing I haven't gone there makes me cry. I feel lucky and privileged to not have taken that first drink. I feel blessed that I am AF and not poisoned with alcohol. I feel happy that I walked myself through the process and made an adult decision not to go there. I feel strong and ready.

Chapter One

July 20, 2013
Day 1
Withdrawal Symptoms.

Yesterday was the first day in as long as I could remember that I didn't take a drink.

Overnight wasn't good. I woke up at 2 a.m. with stomach pains, sure I was going to be sick, shivering and feeling like the flu was imminent, my brain rushing round in circles, and just basically scared witless. I got out of bed at 4 a.m. and sat like a wax dummy in front of a *Deal or No Deal* recording for an hour. I felt like I'd been hit by a train and all my brain was saying was, 'just have a hair of the dog later and you will stop feeling crap'. Last night I thought I was going to go insane knowing there was lager and cider in the fridge and stopping myself having it. My hands were shaking on the second morning, but that was part of the process.

I told my husband I was stopping and he was supportive, although I don't think he understood how badly I was feeling it then. He is a 'normal' drinker in that he just has the odd one when he feels like it. He doesn't crave it so badly by 6 p.m. that violence could happen without it (just joking, but the nerves did get that bad).

I kept telling myself; remember this is normal; this old body is getting rid of all the crap, readjusting to normal settings, so ride it out. Remember to EAT.

It does get easier, they said online. Drink lots of water

during the day and have a nice warm bath before bed to help you to relax. You'll feel so much better soon.

I knew I'd have felt tons worse had I had a drink; I had to remember that. The first few days were always going to be tough, but hang on in there, sister, and it would get better and easier!

On this second day I had already started to cleanse my system and it was bound to hurt for a few hours, then it would be gone; I knew I had to do it at the weekend or else wouldn't do it at all.

They say it takes 72 hours to get alcohol out of the system. But not out of the mind.

I felt like I had a terrible hangover and yet there was no drink in me; in fact I didn't feel that bad when I'd had a drink … no energy, swirling guts, looked like shit …

I kept repeating over and over; just have to see it through and keep thinking about how good it will feel in a few days' time.

Most of that second day, I slept a fair bit, did a lot of walking with the dogs, and by tea time they were both sparked out. The dogs were certainly going to get fitter! The walking kept me sane for several hours without my crutch-in-a-bottle. I had to take heart that I was not alone in trying each day onwards to be alcohol free. I kept myself busy in the house with lots of pointless pottering. I was really very thirsty.

Despite the physical symptoms I actually felt mentally better already, more clear-headed, and my stomach felt empty, rather than full of drink and too much food after getting drink-related munchies as I normally would at the weekend. At the same time of night, around 8 p.m., I would normally be dozing or watching rubbish on the box without taking it in, considering one more drink before bed, and dosing myself with Solpadeine to make sure I got off, even if it meant I knew I would be awake at 3 a.m. I knew the hard bit was still to come.

The odd goings on in my brain and body were OK, just part of the process … the shakes were horrid, but they did pass fairly quickly.

I didn't feel guilty about keeping up those sugar levels; it was a perfect time for indulging in all those naughty but nice treats! Nearly there with the first 3 days … keep going and I wouldn't look back.

I hoped the start of new week would get easier and I didn't allow myself to try too hard to change everything around me.

I had taken every opportunity to wear my middle-aged body out with alcohol, so each day building myself up with a drink was the way to clear the tiredness, fuzzy head, and shaky feelings that came with mini withdrawal. I had to see those symptoms out this time and get over the three-day barrier.

Music playing was lovely and relaxing, and was uplifting. Bath, bed, and light reading worked well. I could still expect the early wake-up, just with no hangover. I spent time writing letters, lists of things to do and reminders, and logging in to the internet.

That evening I had major cravings for sugary drinks or sweets, as my body was craving the sugar that alcohol gave it. I tried not to worry about the feelings; they were normal and would improve. I didn't sleep well again, but sober rest was better rather than drugged-up sleep. Each day completed was a boost to my confidence and self-esteem.

Day 2

The experience of not drinking, even for a few hours, was not easy. I kept questioning my feelings as though I were interviewing someone else, which helped somewhat.

I told a colleague I had decided not to drink 'for a while' (forever seemed too massive) and they said, 'I thought you seemed really quiet, now I know why!' Was this my true character, a miserable bastard? I guessed I seemed quiet because I had a lot to think about. I wondered if the middle of summer was a stupid time of year to stop drinking, but I knew that there was never going to be a perfect time. I was finding I was giving myself a lot of pep talks like that; in the car, at the bathroom mirror, walking to the shops … Trying to convince myself I wasn't making the worst mistake of my life, being as I felt like complete shit. It was important to remember there would be highs as well as lows. I had another bath and an early night, as come night time, being conscious became just too much to bear. The bedtime story I told myself before bed seemed to help:

Once upon a time, there was a beautiful princess called Laurina. On Laurina's eighteenth birthday she was sitting, somewhat sulkily, in a ball gown next to a large lake in the castle grounds. Laurina had already been given many gifts: grace, youth, intellect, and an arse to die for. As she sat wondering what else she could possibly ask for in life, a sneaky, creepy old witch appeared. In her gnarled old witchy hand was a bottle of golden liquid. 'Hello, Laurina,' said the old witch, 'I can see you are conflicted 'cos you actually have everything and a bit more besides, you silly, silly girl, so I have the perfect gift for you. This lovely liquid is called Lambrini, and it makes everything that you have just seem sooo much better. This magic bottle will replenish any time you drink from it. Now, have a swig and don't tell yer Dad.'

'Sounds great,' said Laurina, glugging away.

Many years passed. Laurina attended many lush parties, snogged a lot of frogs, threw up a lot of swan kebabs, and generally prostituted her sense of dignity and self-worth to the ever-overflowing goblet of magical nectar. It didn't matter how many mattresses she had on her four-poster bed – she always slept restlessly. Slowly, the beautiful, vivacious princess began to turn jaded and gnarled – just like the horrid witch who first cast the drink spell upon her.

Then one day – a bit pissed and wobbly – Laurina knocked into the carved oak table which held the magic juice and it spilt and broke – never to replenish again. Laurina was devastated, 'Ooh no, who am I? What about my good-time girl status? How will I manage my courtly duties without the magic juice – NO ONE can do a 'Liz MacDonald on a bender' impression like me!'

But, despite her worried, Laurina managed. It was all OK, and on her thirty-seventh birthday, she got the gift of 'clarity and wisdom', free as she was from the curse of the magic juice. Plus she still had more riches to spend in a major UK Supermarket.

The End.

Day 3
End of day cravings.

I got in from work knackered and the only thing on my mind was getting a drink in me. I felt totally wrung out with the battle inside of not being able to sink my usual and feel that sweet relief of being home and relaxing with a drink … yet I knew the feeling of elation only lasted a short while, then the depression catches up, and the fatigue from work and stress is made worse.

Then there was the interminable dozing on the sofa and not engaging with anyone, living in a trance until bed, then waking up off and on all night. No more of that. I was done with nearly thirty years of that. I was thinking today, as my brain started to wake up, about all the incidents in my life where the Drink Demon, as I thought of it, had taken an opportunity or caused a problem or made me do something risky or thick, and there were literally hundreds of them crowding in.

It was not that I was beating myself up about it, I was just realizing: what the hell have I been doing to myself all these years? All that wasted money and time. But still I thought about a glass of wine and some dark voice said, 'I think one won't hurt.'

I was so thirsty today and no amount of water seemed to quench it. I ate a lot of processed carbs but had no appetite for proper food. Someone online gave good advice about taking vitamins, especially B vitamins, to help with the nerve side of things. The shaky hands had gone, my heart was still fluttering like mad, but I hadn't died! As I mentioned above, I had been drinking way too much, a habit starting where I drank as soon as I got out of school, then got out of university for the day, then when older when I left work for the day, – a nasty habit going on 30 or so years.

I went out and did an hour and half marching the dogs

round the fields; they were in seventh heaven with all the extra exercise. Then I had a major sugar craving which normally I would stifle with a glass of chilled cider, but settled for a hot choc instead before bed. There I was at Day 3 and managing to stick to Coke, tea, and fruit juice.

There were so many thought whizzing around my brain as it came out of the haze, but I was firm with the Drink Demon. I told it to get lost (in slightly firmer terms). Every time I said no to it I felt a little stronger and the Drink Demon's shouting got weaker …

For years I decided to give up every Monday morning but it never lasted – I managed to function, go to work, do chores – but I always felt like an accident waiting to happen.

I needed to change my routine. Instead of flopping out on the sofa with a glass of alcohol, I decided to spend ages watering the garden, take a shower or long bath, and then early to bed with a book. Probably sounds boring but I enjoyed reading chapters and remembering them the next day. Enjoyed painting my nails as I read though all the blogs and inspiring stories online. If I could do it, anyone could. I knew I had to take it a day at a time and be gentle on myself.

Day 4
Lighter physically and mentally.

I was turning into a right hypochondriac with all these aches and pains and hot-flush-type feelings down my legs. I had another hangover-like headache in the morning when I woke up and was sure these symptoms were an actual physical withdrawal. I slept until 5 a.m., which was an improvement, and was thrilled the scales were telling me I was 2 lbs down since starting this journey. On waking I experienced little flutters of excitement at the thought of being in control of my body instead of having the drink dictate how I felt. I found starting the day with the juice of a lemon in hot water helped. I knew my diet needed a complete overhaul, but had no stomach for it at that point.

I kept looking at food during the day and thinking 'urgh', which was a good thing from a slimming point of view, I guessed …

I had the familiar desperate urge to drink as I came in from work that night. The Drink Demon kept saying, 'well, you could do four days off and three days on, how about that as a compromise?' But I knew that before long the Drink Demon would be saying, how about five on two off … big fat no, pal.

By the evening the headache was just starting to subside, and I still felt a little shaky but determined to rid myself of the poison. I went for a walk with my husband along the beach, and I thought, life is looking great. Then yet another bath – baths galore soothed my itchy skin.

Maybe all the aches and pains were there all the time and it was just that I had numbed them with drinking. Consulting the internet told me I was still detoxing, and not to worry about the funny feelings too much, all pretty normal. The flushes (very genteel term, when in fact I sweated like the proverbial pig) and the tingly feelings came and went …

Stick with it, I said to the mirror, drink and rest, eat whatever your body tells you it wants today, give it lots of TLC, and be encouraged that it's nearly over.

Day 5
Jangly nerve thing easing.

Reading other people's stories and advice online gave me such strength because I knew I was not alone. What brave people, to face up to so many difficult issues.

I was still obsessed with my physical symptoms, especially after all the warnings I read about not just stopping drinking as it could be dangerous. I had planned for this by cutting down gradually over about 12 weeks, but it didn't really properly hit me that my stop date was actually the day I decided to have no more drink until the hour actually arrived. God knows how I would have felt if I had just stopped without any cutting down beforehand.

It's true I went through the mill the first three days, but today I was feeling peckish. I also felt a lot more laid back.

The doctor had put me on fluoxetine – I had come to realise the drinking was self-medicating for what this proper medicine now needed to deal with in my head, at least until I felt stronger. The fluoxetine was 10 days in when I had my last drink; I started it knowing I was going to ditch the stuff. The drug was probably contributing to me feeling like shit; hopefully an end was in sight to these symptoms. Either way it was still much better without the booze.

I got a much-needed break from routine because I decided to work from home, so the coming in at 6 p.m. and wanting a drink thing was missed off the list of dodgy moments of the day. My instincts told me to stay busy and make plans, so that the points where I would normally think, oh well, it's late enough to crack open the wine/cider, didn't have a look in.

I gave myself a huge pat on the back for getting this far. The time soon went by as long as I stayed busy, so I knew I could keep with it, even if I felt like climbing up the wall – I was looking forward to feeling better in a few days, and if I thought about it from a working prospective, Monday mornings seemed to whizz around pretty quickly so the weeks would soon slip by.

It struck me that sober people have so many things in common, no matter which part of the world they come from, what language they speak, whether they are short, tall, curvy, thin, religious or not so, from one ethnic group or another, straight or gay – none of that matters when they have common feelings/opinions:

- A desire for change in their lives.
- An interest in how other people change their lives.
- An interest in helping others to change.
- An understanding that things cannot go on as before.
- Curiosity about finding out who they really are and what they are capable of.
- An awareness that drink has inhibited the achievement of goals/potential.
- A realisation that they may not have drunk more than our neighbours, but it was bad enough to make them unhappy and therefore unsustainable as a lifestyle choice.
- A knowledge that they hurt people that they love when they drank.
- A wish to like and be proud of themselves.
- An excitement about what non-drinking could lead to.
- A realisation that being part of a community which values sobriety is a wonderful thing.

Day 6
Trying not to think too far ahead.

This was the longest I had gone drink free since 2009, when I managed 3 months then broke it by celebrating my husband taking redundancy from a job he hated. He just wandered in with two bottles of champagne even though he knew I was trying to give up, only I chose to drink it with him, but I still don't understand why he did that. I guess people without a problem just don't get how slippery our grasp on sanity can be. My husband, bless him, suggested that he kept an eye on me and when he thought I had had enough to drink he would tell me to stop. Well, we had another conversation where I had to explain that I couldn't do that. I couldn't just have a couple of drinks and then leave it. I didn't have that relationship with wine any more, so I was just not going to have the first drink. I didn't blame him for thinking he could help me but I explained that unless a person was going through this themselves, then they couldn't really understand an addict's feelings.

At that moment he was supporting me but kept talking about special events in the future where I could have a drink, and this didn't help. He just didn't get that I could not allow myself to drink again. I, for my part, was making myself block out the thought of never drinking again, because it was far too massive to contemplate.

I did, however, think about events in the future which I knew I would find boring and tedious sober and would normally have a drink to ease the passage, and dreaded them.

When I looked back on my social life, for decades alcohol had always been a central part, and the people around me all drank and would think I was either a snob/ill/weak/not part of the gang any more/mental …

I knew I shouldn't worry about what people thought,

but I supposed they might surprise me.

I had been talking some more to my husband about my decision and he was happy with it. In fact, he said this week I had been wonderful, which surprised me as I thought I was wrecked, and it meant a lot. He said I was not an alcoholic; I was just crap at drinking …

The lengths we go to, first to cover our drinking and then to cover our not drinking! I hadn't dared tell anyone else yet of my decision. I think the point my husband made about choosing friends carefully was a good one; in fact I lost several friends over the years when I tried, fruitlessly, to quit and realised that when I didn't go in the pubs and clubs, some friends were generally very arsey and stopped bothering with me. Nobody needs that kind of 'friendship'.

I spoke openly with my husband and explained that one drink for some is always one drink too many. I told him as time passed I thought I would find that special events wouldn't be boring without booze and that I would actually enjoy (and maybe remember) them more. But, if an event was boring, it would be just as boring when drinking. I thought my husband would also see over time that he could still enjoy special occasions with me whether I drank or not. Let the special occasion be the important thing, not the drink.

There were always going to be difficult occasions – or difficult at first anyway I kept telling myself I was doing so well. I had been invited to a 65th birthday 'do'. It was going to be an all-day thing and although I would know some of the people there, I wouldn't know many. I was going to drive so that took care of that in one sense. I was giving myself a bit of a get out though; if I found it was getting too much, or I was bored, I would be going home at least once during the day (maybe more) to feed the dogs and let them out. I might also spend a lot of time driving around the countryside but it would be a lot better than drinking.

It must be hard for partners, friends, colleagues, and really all people in the lives of drinkers to understand the nature of this addiction.

As for looking into the future with social events, I would just take one day at a time.

I have mentioned that at first my drinking was very socially orientated and a big part of my life for so long and I loved it. It took years of it becoming a worse and worse problem, done at home on the sofa in front of the telly, for it having to go. I had all the usual worries about what people would think of me … maybe one day I wouldn't give a shit and would simply flick my hair defiantly and say , it's my life and I'll live it how I want, like strong people did.

Maybe one day I would get to the point where I actually believed nobody really cared about what actually entered my system and prove to myself it was therefore possible to easily avoid booze if I chose to, at social events.

A friend added: 'Sobriety is worth trying, surely? Being selfish and not thinking about what others think. I made it through a girlie supper last night. I poured everyone wine but poured myself a nice glass of sparkling water in a wine glass and I couldn't believe no one noticed at the dinner table all night. I think people notice (if at all) for a fleeting second! I was dreading last night being boring but I listened to all the gossip, was able to join in without slurring my words, but more importantly was able to give a sensible opinion on this and that which made me feel very much in control.'

Day 7
Friday night bereavement.

I knew Friday night would be the hardest, as it was always my traditional time for downing enough to send me unconscious. I didn't want to come home tonight as I felt I couldn't handle the immense grief I was feeling from about 4 p.m., knowing that my urges would not be satisfied. So I came in with a heavy heart, lay on the bed for an hour feeling sorry for myself and pretending to my OH I was OK. I dropped off and when I woke up I felt much better.

I got a glass of sparkling water with ice and made a very spicy chili. I could say sitting there that I actually was doing Friday night as a sober person. I was astonished and proud, and relieved. I hoped if I had trigger points that weekend I'd manage to see them through. Week two started the next day.

A friend told me about her Friday night: 'Coming in from the pub, having been there since 7 p.m., I counted three pints of lime and soda water. I left my companions hammered … thanking God I would not have their heads in the morning. I was able to drive home too; a first. Here's to more nights like that; I'm actually looking forward to tomorrow. Usually I'll wake up on the sofa the next day when it's going dark, knowing I'll spend the day trying not to bite people's heads off due to nerves and just waiting for a so-called 'civilised' time to get a hair of the dog and feel better, thus ruining Sunday as well.'

The expectation that the week has to be rounded off with alcohol was one that I had come to accept as written. Here was another milestone and another good habit forming. I kept thinking how good I would feel the next day.

I used to be literally seconds away from drinking from

most Friday afternoon onwards, had to battle with it for hours while trying to run my training session and be professional, when I was just a mess inside. I comforted myself with the thought that I was not alone and I could do this if others could; I had this time recognised the trigger and next Friday I would be ready for it and have a plan in place. If I could do 7 more days of the second week I could push it further next time and see this first horrendous week as just a practice.

When I was up tomorrow walking the mutts in the early sunshine (or rain, I didn't care) and feeling strong, I would be also be stopping to give myself a metaphorical smug hug.

Day 8
Into week 2 and dealing with a new routine.

Last weekend I was high on the excitement of giving up, and it was all novel and different. As the days went on the reality of what I had decided started to hit home and culminated in the middle of last night/early morning with a proper grieving session for how things used to be. Of course the Drink Demon had only good memories to remind me about and conveniently forgot to mention the nasty stuff, of which I was so ashamed and horrified, knowing that I had it in me to sink so low, so many times.

When I thought of what I gave away for a drink and a supposedly good time over the years, and how I allowed myself to be used, I wanted to weep buckets. I did indeed cry tears of pure self-pity.

Now I was not drinking I was faced just with myself, with no distractions. I didn't even know whether I liked myself or who I was. I had just drifted through life without a plan and spent all my time reacting to situations, rather than making adult decisions about my future.

Please don't think this was a woe is me thought process – I was actually pleased to be having those sober thoughts, pleased to be thinking about the big stuff. A couple of weekends ago I would be sitting there focusing on how to alleviate my bad head, swirling guts, and skin oozing stale drink and that would be as far as I got, in fact my decision would be to have a drink that night (meaning early afternoon) and deal with stuff 'tomorrow', whenever that may be. It was always 'tomorrow'. Now I had a fighting chance of sorting my life out. I felt like I was becoming a different person, quite a bizarre feeling at my age, but good. Life really was different out of the haze.

Reading stories online, I found it amazing that there were just so many of us out there, all thinking and feeling the same.

I had more little indulgent sobs. I hadn't ever written down or said any of this stuff and it sounded so mental when I read my journal back; I kept thinking, get a grip, woman! I had to be proud of this new strength and get some self-esteem from working hard to get through it. Hang in there, I told myself. It gets better.

I had already got to the point where the novelty had started to wear off and I thought today, is this it? But I somehow got through it, and the excitement returned. It would get easier, I promised myself for the hundredth time. I had never stopped for this long and never thought I could or would. It was scary.

A friend wrote: 'One of the best descriptions I have read was the washing machine in the head: trying to get rid of alcohol first, then the stains it leaves – sometimes very black – and that process in our head is tough. I add "the spin-dryer effect". Gradually the sinking feeling is fading and other good thoughts are allowed to enter.

I may not get many more chances again to wash my head out, so I hang in for what it's worth. Small, but good things keep happening to me, and I hold my head up a little higher each day.'

Day 9
Weird dreams.

I wondered if other people had been having strange dreams as part of their withdrawal. I can't remember the last time I slept well enough to dream, or at least remember them, but they had been coming back in recent days. Last night I dreamed that I was pouring bottle after bottle of wine down the sink, and when I woke up today I felt such relief and calmness.

My dreams, if I had them when drinking, used to be mainly be either getting chased by a vicious dog, or being lost in a strange city, or having to go to the toilet in a public place with people walking past. Back then I would wake between 3 and 4 a.m., anxious and sweaty from the get-go. But today I was tranquil and free. Another dream I remembered from my sober sleep was of finding myself as drunk as I had been in previous days. When I woke I was so relieved at finding myself still sober.

Day 10
Saying the words out loud.

Some very brave and honest people had been posting online about how they were starting to see the reality of their relationships with different people and what seemed to be changing and it made me think about my own.

A friend commented, ‘I wondered, when I was out with my folks yesterday, why I couldn’t tell them I have decided not to drink any more, and why I copped out when asked why I refused a drink; I said I was driving. I wonder why I don’t trust my friends to say “I am a non-drinker now”. I wonder also why I doubted that my OH would be pleased and happy that I am happy – I do feel lucky in this respect reading some other experiences. I talked to him at length yesterday because he did ask, “Is this definitely it?”, and it felt really strange actually saying it out loud for the first time, because up until now I have only written about it.’

I could honestly say that whilst the opportunity to tell many friends that I had given up hadn’t presented itself yet, that I was proud and would be proud to announce my decision. It was not about them, it was about me. No hangovers, no memory loss, no drink driving, more stable hormones, and the rest.

This time around, however, many of my family knew I had decided to become AF by the fact that I looked less worn-out, so I didn’t have to explain or make excuses. I had so far come out more to friends than family, and realised that they had a past too, not always a drunken one, but who hasn’t some shame of doing something wrong in their life? Of course there are those who like to appear perfect and won’t admit they ever sinned. I did before on several previous AF attempts say to many ‘never again, I don't drink any more'. Now I was using the words, 'I don't want a drink now or today, so I'll have a sparkling cranberry.'

Another friend added: 'I tried beating around the bush with it at first. You don't want to say it out loud because you don't have confidence that you can do it, and if they see you drinking again they may say, "wow she really does have a problem if she can't even stop". I have to say I've had two completely negative responses from very good old friends … They don't think I have a drink problem but I think by accepting the fact that I do would be also admitting that they do. I've only told one other friend; a 30-year-long friendship who didn't question how much I had been drinking, but said she totally understood why I didn't want to drink, since she'd witnessed the negative effects it had on me many times. I have to admit that I didn't actually tell her how much I had been drinking. I didn't want to be told that it wasn't a problem; that could be used as an excuse to drink again.'

How does it feel to say it out loud and make it real to yourself? Serious, I would say. No more denial; committed. I resolved only to tell those who needed to know at first, until I had confidence in myself. These were the people that knew I had a problem anyway so probably didn't count. I shied away from really 'telling' anyone else. It would just sort of happen and I didn't think it was anybody else's business anyway, so wouldn't go out of my way to explain. Anyone who cared for me was going to be pleased and supportive. Only the ex-drinker will know when and if they want to tell people. I would wait till I had got a bit more confidence. There was no rush.

Day 11

Making myself stick to new routines.

The big thing I was finding with this AF malarkey was the need to have plans in place rather than allowing myself to sink back into the rut that made me rely on a bottle or a can most nights. Here they are:

Morning – take antidepressant, longer walk with pooches, shower, and drive.

Day – work and try not to eat too much sugar despite constant hypo/light-headed feeling which only sugar seems to stop (working on it).

Afternoon – drive home, fight cravings, rehearse driving past supermarket, play loud music, get in feeling shit, loll about on bed feeling like a wreck and arguing with addict voice in head (about an hour).

Tea time – cook proper meal, go on the internet to talk to other ex-drinkers and stay on through night, drink water, tea.

Evening – long walk with pooches, bed by 10, read or watch bit of telly, sleep by 10.30.

This sounded horrifically boring when I wrote it down as I was literally doing the same thing every day, but at that moment it was keeping me sane. I wondered if anyone else had any new routines they needed to stick to in order to keep them steady. Or was I the most boring person in the world? On the subject of boring, I wasn't exactly the most interesting person when I was swigging vino every night.

My OH kindly brought home 6 bottles of San Pellegrino sparkling water and fresh orange juice tonight so I swigged fizzy orange, which filled me up and was so much nicer than alcohol. Alcohol didn't really taste that good in the first place, being as it's a poison and that …

I was really craving sweet stuff – I didn't expect that. I had a lovely glass of ginger beer after the fizzy orange and I drank lime and lemon before bed. I had to stick to a routine – it was working for me and that was all that mattered.

I played patience obsessively on my computer and also played the boardgame *Othello* for hours on the app on my phone. Now the brain fog was clearing I could sit in one place long enough to read and was starting to read books again (where did that habit go?) but it was back. It was like becoming a new person (or the original without drink).

The one thing that was right on time every day was the Drink Demon's voice – totally out of the blue: 'Oooh, wouldn't a nice glass of wine be good about now?' I was finding it a lot easier to push them aside though, and was instead looking forward to a nice cup of herbal tea and the (now obligatory) Dairy Milk bar. Sort out the Sugar Monster was next on the 'to do' list.

These first few weeks were for me about establishing a safe routine; if or when I started to think, 'Hmmm, this is a bit boring', I would know I needed to mix it up a little. I wasn't yet ready for any AF nights out. It was hard, not because I wanted to drink (I didn't), but because I didn't know if I'd be the same person out without booze.

I also had to research some things that I might enjoy to fill in the enormous gaps of time which were previously filled with drinking, thinking about drinking, and recovering from drinking. I was supposedly a bright enough individual. I was sure I could come up with some.

I decided in the very early days it was good to keep things really simple and practise KISS (keep it simple, sober). As I started to physically feel better and my energy levels improved (as well as my self-esteem) I would naturally feel a bit more inclined to do more things. I wouldn't always want to go to bed at 9 p.m. and read *Harry Potter* books … surely not?

But I did need to benefit from a quieter life for a bit. In the past I was always dashing and doing a lot of socialising as well as working. One thing was for sure, I was going to have the fittest dogs in the country. They didn't know what on earth had happened with all these extra and longer perambulations, but they certainly weren't complaining about all the bonus exercise.

Day 12
Gardening.

One of the things that kept me sober these last few days had been my little allotment (vegetable garden). Our flat came with a 'garden' which was basically an overgrown patch of land with rickety fencing around three sides and none at the front, so local dog owners frequently let their dogs relieve themselves on it.

Getting a fence across the front put a stop to that business, and I propped up the most rickety bits of fence by really hammering in the loosest of the posts, which was a very satisfying exercise, especially if I considered that the posts could well be someone's head; more strength to my elbow in that respect.

The next thing to do was sort out the overgrown hawthorn hedge at the back of the garden which took up about six feet more space than it was entitled to. A kind neighbour lent me a pair of those big secateurs with long arms and I pruned away for a day or so, until a huge pile of spiky branches sat in the middle of the site. This evening I had a big fire of as much debris as I could find. I love outdoor fires, and this ceremonial burning seemed to set the scene for literally and metaphorically setting new boundaries in my life. I had loads more room at the end of my garden and already more room in my recovering mind.

I couldn't find anything else to burn, rather disappointingly, so planned to set about clearing the huge tangles of nettles, brambles, and random weeds, as well as deeply entrenched tufts of grass growing up to my waist in parts. I was finding all sorts during this stage – a tiny horse shoe which was probably from a pit pony, as we lived in a row of former pit cottages, an engine plate dated 1939 which a neighbour said would have been from an army vehicle, lots of animal teeth (horse or pony probably), a very rusty dog choker chain, an old garden gate hidden under layers of grass, some strange steel tubing wrapped in bubble plastic, and an animal feed bag, which I suspected was a gun before I unwrapped it, but who knows why it had been buried. Lovely blisters acquired, even with gloves. The allotment and all the hard physical work was keeping me away from thoughts of drinking, especially in the evenings and at weekends.

Gardening neighbours had left me plants to go in, and it was such a delight to wake up this morning and look out the window to see a little of tray of seedlings on the allotment path, waiting to be planted. I am so lucky to have amazing, warm-hearted neighbours.

My recovery was helped so much by this project and by the people who had time to stop and speak.

I could thoroughly recommend this type of outdoor activity as a distraction from booze – even if you grow things in a welly or a tyre.

Day 13
Feeling a strange thing I'm calling elation.

Tomorrow I would reach a fortnight off booze. Although I still felt like I had been run over by a tank every morning, there was a period during the day where I got a tingle of ecstasy when I thought about being a non-drinker. I would describe it as extreme happiness of a kind I could only remember experiencing a few times on special occasions. It was a bit like what I thought I would feel if I ever won the lottery. It only lasted a few seconds but the feeling was so intense and such a sense of pride and achievement came over me that I was willing to put up with all the exhaustion caused by fighting the drink just to have it.

I was still a long way off being comfortable with not drinking, and it occupied a good slice of my thinking, but I could start to see a time on the horizon when I would be comfortable with being AF. At that moment I was not safe enough to be able to set myself on a sober pedestal, or polish my halo too often. Mostly it was in a drawer.

Although I had a lot of times when I was feeling a bit down, I was still in a better place without the poison. I didn't exactly wake up bouncing each morning, but thought that, well, at least I woke up having slept without a drink in me. It was a novelty not to have a hangover and to be without the angst-ridden fears that followed me everywhere for years. I remembered going to bed, what I ate and drank and did, instead of having to look for clues. I knew I could face whatever the day brought. I still got incredibly strong emotions, memories, and feelings hitting me at the most unexpected times. I still got overwhelmed by the sheer massiveness of the change in my life … and I was so grateful. Hopefully the tank that ran me over every night in my sleep would turn into a little car soon.

I woke up with a new cold sore and the same old flu-type feeling, but hey ho – I was free of drink and would get through this. I was crying a lot too, at the most inconvenient times, but still hanging in there.

The lousy feelings that came with the struggle some days were very tough, but then when I got the little uplifting feelings of hope I noticed how far I had actually come. There were plenty of times before when I'd struggled and then thought I was getting better, so of course I was cured and could drink moderately. I lost sight of the fact I was addicted to numbing my feelings; the buzz, the high and yet the low, washed-out hangover was the only realistic result in the end of my worst drinking days. This AF attempt I would not run to, or use, alcohol to hide my feelings or myself.

A wise poster online talked about 'Feel, Deal, Heal'. Suddenly I had all the feelings and emotions that I used to numb coming back. I was definitely feeling! It could be overwhelming at times, but the tears were good. I needed to feel these feelings properly for the first time in ages, let them come and acknowledge them, then let them go as I heal. Feel, Deal, Heal.

This 13 days AF was one of the proudest achievements of my life. It was a great feeling and it was real.

Day 14
The second dry Friday was better.

This time last week I was a pitiful wreck rolling about on my bed and feeling self-indulgently glum; quite pathetic really, all for the sake of a poison.

The drive home tonight I thought about it less and wanted it less, and the Friday-night tradition of getting plastered and spoiling the weekend seemed less attractive … really could not think why I wouldn't be missing spending a load of cash, getting diverticulitis again, annoying my partner, ageing my body, depressing my mind, piling on excess weight, hating the world and myself, wasting some more precious time …

I was a useless dancer but I felt like having a dance or two, clicking those heels, being daft, and most of all saying a great big GET STUFFED to the drink. How naughty was I.

Others at the same stage were feeling the same: 'I had a friend over for the evening, we cooked a nice meal, drank soft drinks, did face packs and nail varnish. Proper girlies. I was looking forward to enjoying the lovely morning which was coming my way. I felt great that I was already looking back and questioning why I ever drank. I had to carry that forward and be strong.

Despite the cold sore enhancing my lip and the ever-present light-headed flu feeling, I dared to say I was feeling drunk with relief and happiness; either that or the fluoxetine was starting to kick in.

Day 15
Annoyingly cheerful.

My good mood was continuing. I kept questioning the feeling and thinking, 'You do realise something terrible will happen shortly,' but that was the addict talking. The sly Drink Demon voice that said, 'Well, missy, since everything really will go wrong, because it always does, you may as well anticipate it and have a bloody drink.'

'Well actually, Drink Demon,' I said, 'I'm just going to be a bit different today and take it as it comes. So take your negative thinking, your finger prodding, and your told-you-so whining voice and stick it where the sun don't shine. Cheers.'

When bad or difficult things happened, I was sober, I had more emotional resources and emotional capacity to think problems through, and, to a certain extent, could choose how to react or respond. Now I still made mistakes and acted like a prat on occasion, but I felt more authentic in myself, as I truly owned my emotions most of the time. Very subtle, but life-changing coping mechanisms.

I was finding that the advice I was given to keep a journal of my recovery, get all the feelings and emotions down on paper, handwritten or typed, was a very necessary part of my healing and moving on. I couldn't function without my journal.

I looked back at old diaries and there were a lot of blanks for each year of drinking. I was really enjoying writing down the good new days that had arrived for me, but not forget the trials, too, that I hoped to surmount in the future. Here was another new project, one of many, but one that, for once, would work.

I actually felt quite scared that I felt good whilst others who related their stories online were feeling bad and thought maybe I was doing something wrong and that it was all going to crash spectacularly for me, like every time before … but it hadn't so far. I felt this was the last try. I'd found hope and a whole new happy me I'd forgotten about.

I decided it was a good plan to take today easy and slow and nice things would happen, without me beating myself up because I was tempted – and I still did not give in. The voice moved around with me during the day but would not last more than few seconds. Today my mantra was 'Got a lot of living to do' and catch-up time was starting to be so important to me. Goodbye to the old drinking ways and in with the new non-alco me.

Keep dancing.

Day 16
There is always a reason to drink.

Reading blogs from people who still drank and recognising your own drinking self in their experiences was extremely poignant. I knew these 'reasons' to drink didn't cut it for me any more.

But I supposed the other side of blogging, reading, and trying to work out my own reasons for why I effed up so badly was that hearing the same stuff from so many people who were convinced they were OK, when they patently weren't, was really tricky. I desperately wanted to get them by the shoulders and give them a damn good shake. Of course, they would think I was nuts.

The Drink Demon tells you that you can't give drink up until after your holiday, or until after that wedding, or until your flu clears up. Because, after the holiday or the flu or the wedding, there would be yet another reason why it didn't make sense to give up; there would always be a reason. That's how I lived for 30 years, making up reasons why I couldn't shake it. As I said, I was such a bloody long way from being able to preach to anyone about how to live, but as someone who had put off and put off for literally decades, I wanted to think I could make just one procrastinator stop and wonder how they actually sounded.

The Drink Demon always played twatful games with my head. Much easier to be FREE.

I wasn't sure if I was being a bit harsh on myself but some things needed saying. I had done all the 'reasons' and ended up here, pretty much wrecked. I didn't think I had to call myself an alcoholic or label myself in any way, I just had to think, was this stuff making me happy and healthy, and if not, then it was time to get rid. So that's what I did.

Day 17
Reading, reading, reading.

I was increasingly interested in what other people did to get through this situation and was reading avidly, including authors such as Jason Vale and Lucy Rocca and Sarah Turner, who co-wrote *The Sober Revolution*. Reading and learning from others was my salvation at that point and I was feeling less alone for it. Reading was such an important way to stay positive and looking forward, whatever I could get hold of. It was a great way to fill in the wine time. All the books and blogs were best seen as a tool. Everything I read made me look at alcohol in a new way.

Like anything else, the resources out there were so numerous … reading helped me stay on track, but it was just one tool in my tool case, nothing more, nothing less. Even if I did not agree with everything I read, I decided to just focus on what worked for me.

That night I watched the movie *Flight* with Denzel Washington. It was about a pilot who skilfully managed to save 96 lives in a crash landing when he was drunk. It was definitely good material if anyone wanted some aversion therapy.

I was making notes obsessively to try and straighten out in my head the reasons for carrying on 'doing sobriety'. For anyone doing the same, it might be helpful to write out your own list.

1. I hate myself when I consort with the Drink Demon.
2. Other sober people dislike/hate me when I even speak to it.
3. I have ruined too many situations by hanging out with it and its buddies.
4. I have ruined too many relationships for the same reason (it is so possessive, it hates me having other friends/relationships).

5. I sleep badly after a night with it; all the things it said and did fuck with my mind.

6. I eat badly when I'm with it.

7. My guts turn inside out when I spend time with it.

8. I put weight on even going near it.

9. I look like shit when I let it help with my hair and make-up, but without make-up I am flushed and sweaty-looking.

10. People laugh at me (not with me unless they are also pissed) when I sit with it.

11. I waste money because I never get it back.

12. I waste time trying to keep up with it.

13. I am always thirsty when I drink with it.

14. I am embarrassed when I drink in its company.

15. I am embarrassing when I drink in its company.

16. I forget my priorities when it gets in my head.

17. I break the law or encourage others to do so when I associate with it.

18. I hurt my loved ones when I put the Drink Demon first.

19. I damage my liver when I get involved in its world.

20 I also risk breast cancer when I drink (and stomach, bowel, kidney, bladder, throat, and mouth cancer).

21. I also put too much strain on my heart.

22. I also risk a life-destroying stroke.

223. People don't trust me when I spend time with the Drink Demon.

24. I cannot afford the things I like when I give the Drink Demon my money instead.

25. I ruin holidays when I take it with me.

26. I cannot make love properly when it insists on being in the room with us; completely off-putting.

27. I lose myself when it pisses off and leaves me.

28. It encourages me to say dumb stuff because it is amused by this.

29. I shorten my life when I take risks on our nights

out.

30. I hurt children when I show I prefer it to them.

31. I am moody when I am with it and when I am missing it.

32. The house looks like a tip after it's been round.

33. My personal hygiene goes to pot when I engage with it.

34. I develop yet more bad habits when I follow its example.

35. I instantly want to smoke when I see it.

36. I spend money on cigarettes I cannot afford when I meet up with it.

37. I buy pointless comfort purchases and crap from catalogues because it encourages me.

38. I make excuses when I want to be with it.

39. I am in denial when I let it influence me.

40. I can always find another shit excuse to spend time with it.

41. I am expecting someone else to be responsible for me when I hook up with it.

42. I put myself in danger when I opt for its company.

43. I also injure myself, often ending up poorly on the sofa or in A&E.

44. I also associate with low-quality people.

45. People also take advantage of me in its company.

46. I also dumb myself down.

47. I do not develop/progress intellectually or emotionally when it's in the room.

48. I cannot help others when I am stuck with the Drink Demon.

49. I am selfish and self-centred just like it when I drink.

50. I take crazy risks when we are out together.

51. I create bad memories just from being with it.

52. I can never move on while it is pissing in my lug.

53. People disrespect my body when I am otherwise

engaged with it.

54. People also think it is OK to hurt me.

55. Men can also sexually abuse me.

56. Men can also hit me/call me names with free rein and blame my drinking for their behaviour.

57. I cannot remember who is to blame when I row with the Drink Demon.

58. I cannot remember what happened to my body when I was with it.

59. I deprive the emergency services/the taxpayer of money when I put money in its pocket instead.

60. I spend too much time being ill when I take it in.

61. I cannot be arsed to keep fit when it is trying to divert my attention.

62. I neglect my pets when I spend all my time with it.

63. I put off doing life when I'm out with it.

64. I miss out on happy times when I listen to it.

65. I blame others for my mistakes and am encouraged to do so by it.

66. I miss the beautiful sunrise and the sunset when I am sat talking to it.

67. I suppress my personality when I let it dominate me.

68. I spend too much time in bed after my showdowns with it.

69. I create wrinkles and skin like a scarlet rhino's backside when I listen to its advice.

70. My face/expression looks like the back end of a cow/ a twice-dropped pie when I wake up the morning after a night with it.

71. I make other people miserable when I neglect them to be with it.

72. I lose the power of rational thought when I believe its stuff.

73. I am telling young, impressionable people it is OK to get pissed when I spend so much time with it.

74. I lose friends/family when I ignore them and their needs and go out with it instead.

75. I feel guilty when I am with it.

76. People think I am strange because I am obsessed with it.

77. Drinking with the Drink Demon ultimately makes me lonely.

78. I mistake the Drink Demon for a friend when I drink.

79. My judgment in most areas is skewed when I listen to its advice.

80. I make ridiculous statements like 'I haven't reached rock bottom yet – that's when I will stop' when I am in conversation about it.

81. I put everyone and everything second to drink when I get its call.

82. I am not safe and neither are my family when I let it in my house.

83. I force others to be my carers when I am temporarily or permanently disabled by the Drink Demon.

84. I talk utter shit when I am with it.

85. People think I am thick when I talk about it as a friend.

86. I cannot let my creative side blossom when I play second fiddle to the Drink Demon.

87. I cannot remember what my creative side even is when I am with it.

88. I do not know who I am/what I am really like when I have it in my head.

89. I cannot get even with people, put them in their place, or prove I am right when I am shackled to the Drink Demon.

90. I cannot show people I am as strong and important as them when I am being dominated by it.

91. I cannot love properly the people who need my love when I give all my love to it.

92. I will always have dirty secrets held by it to blackmail me.

93. I behave like an animal when I party with it.

94. I became a drug addict when I took it in.

95. I spend all my time wanting to stop seeing it after I first agreed to see it.

96. I weaken other people's resolve not to engage with it when I drink too.

97. I am not contributing to society when I take it into my confidence.

98. I am allowing supermarkets to continue to strangle the life out of small communities when I let it call the shots.

99. I am not helping the environment when I let it influence me.

100. I am a right twatful pain in the ass when I spend time with it.

Day 18
Finally got a night's sleep.

Relieved and happy to report I slept all night which was fantastic for me after hardly getting any since packing in the drink. Most mornings I had been waking up feeling worse than when I was drinking; dry mouth, headache, aching body, generally feeling like I'd had at least a bottle of wine. But this morning I actually felt 'normal' (whatever that was).

That morning in my happy little state, I started thinking about all the friendly language that people use around drink. They call it a 'snifter' and a 'tipple' and lots of cutesy words, and I've done that myself too. Time for 'drinkies', 'wine o'clock', 'hot toddy', and so on. Subconsciously it was a way for some people to tell themselves what they were doing was not that bad. I believed the nonsense people spouted about the heady aromas in wine, the lemon and the honey and all that daftness, like it was an art form. Just think about a liver riddled with yellow fat and great big holes caused by the alcohol literally rotting it and then consider if drinking excessively is an art form.

The morning 'alcohol-free hangovers' were a pain but I had to persevere. I hoped I managed to shake them off soon. It was a disappointment to realise I was not automatically going to sleep like a baby once the drink wore off, but the Drink Demon was so big and strong, saying 'ooh, a little drink will send you off, why not try it … ' No, no, no I had to make myself too clever to fall for that. I wanted a healthy liver more than a cheeky glass of Prosecco.

I read about something called Post-Acute Withdrawal Syndrome (PAWS), which can last for up to two years. NOT what I wanted to hear. But, at least a plausible reason for me feeling so low, lacking in energy, and not sleeping.

It could make you feel so bad that you began to think 'one little drink would perk me up' But after having read as much as I could about PAWS … one little drink was NOT the answer. Sticking with it and taking things easy was the way to handle things.

A friend concurred: 'I was fortunate that having had a liver-function test I know it is not damaged through years of over indulging, but I certainly don't want to get to the point where it is. Quit while I am ahead. The liver is an amazing organ and can repair itself if people stop drinking, more severe liver damage won't heal, but it can be halted in its progression. I visualise my liver as a nice shiny purply-red colour because I have stopped drinking. I thought maybe I expected to be feeling fab every day, but of course life isn't like that, even sober life. Life is life and takes a toll on our bodies and minds in many other ways. So the crappy, tired days still come, interspersed with slightly more energetic ones. We have to learn to go with the flow and accept every day for how it is, and be patient.'

Day 19
Working from home (on me).

I had to work from home today after another rubbish night's sleep and waking up feeling like I'd been on the town all night. Wished I could shake this. Not sure what was going on as mentally I felt great, but this old and tired body was just not staying with the programme. For many years I had abused and tormented it, and now I was expecting a lot of it. I needed to go lie on a beach for a fortnight.

The books and blogs I was reading daily continued to interest and irritate at the same time. So many times people talked about not considering themselves to have a drink problem if they could go AF all week then just get stuck in at the weekends. That was me for years. This behaviour was not I was in control, but because I had so many restrictions placed on my life during the week to stay functional that I deluded myself I was coping; but actually I was still an addict, just binge drinking within restrictions. After many years, even the restrictions didn't matter. It was a 'progressive' illness all right.

I felt brave at work yesterday, casually dropping the info in a lunchtime chat that I hadn't drank for nearly three weeks, and got lots of surprised looks – not directed specifically at me because no one there knew I had a problem with it – but just the idea of not drinking for that 'long'. What a funny old world. Stay strong.

I was pleased that for the most part my journal sounded so strong and positive. It was good to read it back to myself, and made me pick myself up and shake myself down. I couldn't do AF without my daily journal.

I guessed the good and bad days would come in waves. Sometimes I was full of energy and could not sit still and other times like today I just wanted to put my head under the duvet. That was life, and it was sober. Life didn't become magically wonderful, it just become life. It would take a while to adjust to the emotional ups and downs when I had been numbing myself for so many years.

I started to feel angry with the alcohol and tobacco industries. What giants us ordinary 'little' people faced, and all these poor children and young people being targeted from such a young age, with advertising for drink everywhere I looked. How could most people ever beat the brainwashing? But I had to keep believing it could be done.

I didn't want to be a marketing victim. I was starting to hate the multi-billion pound/dollar industry that pushes a dangerous addictive substance and hooks young kids. I didn't let the tobacco industry get me and I was not going to let the booze industry get me either. I would stick with it.

I was feeling much better but still very tired. I had been waking up bright and bushy tailed any time between 4 a.m. and 6 a.m., but today I was fighting to drag myself out of bed when the alarm went off. I reckoned this was normal. I was hoping it passed. But despite the short hours of sleep I was happy and feeling like this was the best thing I had done for me in a bloody long time.

I loved the passage in Jason Vale's book *Kick the Drink Easily* where he explained about how it would look if we said we said we weren't addicted to bananas – only had them at weekends and maybe one day during the week. At the very least we tried to have two banana-free days a week. This brought the stupidity of addiction to alcohol home to me.

I thought having the alcoholic label can be crippling for some people who already have low self-esteem; the more I developed my own thinking on the subject of addiction the less inclined I was to attach one single diagnosis to everyone's situation and I concluded everyone is capable of amazing achievements whatever their individual circumstances. Calling yourself an alcoholic can be as damaging as having the habit in the first place, because then you start to compare yourself with other 'alcoholics', and then the Drink Demon jumps in and says, 'Oh, you're not as bad as any of them, ergo you haven't got a problem and you aren't actually alcohol-dependent at all.' Ergo carry on drinking in your 'modest' fashion. So wrong!

With the continuing flu like symptoms, I kept thinking that this was ridiculous, and I could not possibly have alcohol still in my system, but I thought the mental effects would take a lot longer to shift, and I knew the effect my thinking had on my physical wellbeing. It was also possible the fluoxetine was disrupting my sleep, but I was liking being on it and was willing to put up with less sleep for the bigger benefits during my waking hours.

Overall, though, I was so enjoying each day and inspiring myself to keep strong by trying to be positive. My sleep returning would be the icing on the alcohol-free cake.

Being honest with myself about past delusion and self-inflicted restrictions on drinking helped me recognise why over recent years my drinking had worsened. When restrictions were loosened I always consumed more, hence the weekend bingeing.

I was starting to see myself, perhaps arrogantly, as a pioneer. Certainly I recognised I was one of these stubborn people where the more I was told something wasn't possible, the more I wanted to do it.

Reading as widely as possible continued to really open my eyes to the way people are conned about the fun, glamour, and acceptability of booze as part of sophisticated marketing that is both relentless and shameless.

Day 20
Considering what toxic means.

One of the interesting and weird things I found about packing in the drink was the way my taste buds and general food preferences changed, and the way I thought about some things (and people) as toxic. I felt virulent about it. Alcohol actually frightened me. I bought some Bavarian alcohol-free lager and had a bottle of it that night, but I was surprised how scared I felt of drinking it and kept checking the label to make sure I wasn't making a mistake. It was a bit like a vegetarian eating a meat-free sausage. Plus it tasted pretty yuk, but then alcoholic drinks do really unless mixed with something else, or chilled to the point where you cannot taste them anyway.

As far as food went, I couldn't explain it but I had gone right off sandwiches, which I used to love, but now the thought of soggy bread and limp fillings made me feel nauseous. Biscuits I craved along with crisps.

With people, there some that I now regarded as toxic and thanked God they were out of my life, and I wished I had never let them near me in the first place. They would never hurt me again. I was so proud of my husband for his concern and his support and for being my best friend. Anyone who was not absolutely delighted for someone doing this needed to have their motives questioned, I felt.

It was quite an emotional rollercoaster to be on. I alternated between anger and bitterness, and total happiness and optimism. I had hung round with such low-quality people over the years because of my drinking and was trying not to beat myself up about all the time I'd wasted, but it was hard not to. I supposed I was starting to have a bit of a life laundry; I didn't want to fill my body with alcohol or spend hours in bars talking rubbish any more. On the one hand I felt relieved and excited to be doing different things, but on the other I was a bit sad that I wasted so much time with the wrong people, behaving like a muppet and achieving so very little. I decided to get stuck into my job properly, do some studying and try new things and most of the 'new' me was a result of getting alcohol out of my life. How amazing was that?

It was time to really feel what was right for me, going forward – people, food, drinks, places, everything. It was time to give the toxic and negative stuff a wide berth.

Day 21
Three weeks down … it's been emotional.

I was fighting a lot of demons. It was our wedding anniversary at the weekend and we were getting taken out for a meal, but I felt terrible because I didn't want to go; it was going to be too scary not drinking. I literally wanted nothing to do with anything that reminded me of drinking. Even people talking about still doing drinking made me feel anxious.

I still felt angry with myself for wasting so much of my life, with low quality people in low-quality places and doing low-quality things that wasted my precious life and gave away so much of myself to people, who didn't deserve my time, or my company. I was angry with my childhood for not giving me the self-confidence and pride to think more of myself and treat myself better, or prepare me for life ahead. I felt angry with myself for despite being well-educated and with half a brain I had not had the wit to see what I was doing and wasting, by getting wasted.

At the same time I felt enormous pride and satisfaction for getting the magic three weeks under my belt. I felt stronger than ever, as long as I was allowed to stay in my comfort zone. I was reluctant to come out of it just then, until I could form an opinion about how I wanted my boundaries to be.

I found in recent days that food actually tasted better sober. Also, having never been a regular consumer of soft drinks (juice was only for breakfast), I switched to fizzy water with ice, which felt a bit more exciting than still water, mixed with a bit of lime or apple juice if I wanted to add a bit more flavour.

When I came in tonight I was half prepared to have to start drinking again, but reading and keeping my journal kept me away from the booze. I decided to take all that pride and satisfaction, get made up, and go out celebrate our anniversary. I planned what I would be drinking with my meal. I wanted to be AF; I was AF, and life continued AF.

Chapter Two

Day 22
Memories resurface
£60,000 and 4 stone.

I had been blogging relentlessly since the start of this journey and it saved me – I had just got a lot to get off my chest and getting it written down felt like a release.

The other thing I started computing while staring at the ceiling in the dark was how much money I had actually peed down the toilet (or back lanes). I reckoned alcohol alone came to just under £30k over 28 years and that was a conservative estimate based on a low average of £80 a month. (I was always pretty good at bumming free drinks off people too but hadn't counted that). Added to that was getting into places to drink, buying nice clothes/make-up/hair to go get pissed up (important to look 'nice' even when staggering round the streets), cigarettes which I always puffed on like a fourteen-year-old when drunk, taxis as too drunk to drive, drink-related junk food, hangover food the next day, painkillers, lost pay/sackings from 'sick' days caused by hangovers, buying unnecessary treats to try to forget drinking incidents, and so on … add another conservative £30k.

Then there was the 4 stone I gained over that period, which I was now losing fast, thank God. Not because I was on a diet as such, but because I was moving my body more and roughly 8000 drink calories a week were no longer causing a host of health problems. I was hydrating properly and despite the new biscuit habit was eating much better. I thought about post-drinking session pizzas and kebabs and wanted to puke, frankly.

My guy was amazing and he was my strength, but I was also starting to feel I also had my inner strength to get through this, one day at a time.

My journal/blogs made me feel less alone than when I drank. Only honesty and acceptance could take me forward, but people responded to me online in such a kind way and it made me feel like I had a whole new set of friends. My scenario was one that thousands went through.

I thought of all the years all the bargain offers of 3 bottles of wine for £10 and 8 cans of cider for a fiver, that I felt so clever buying, yet never saved me money because I just drank it quicker and it cost me my health, which is invaluable.

I was aware – being, as I was, only a few weeks old as it were – that I was very much in a honeymoon phase with alcohol-free life and so my journal had been up to now largely peppered with upbeat comments about the joys of being sober. Of course, there was a very sad and dark side to the last 30 years that I had been drinking and these stories and feelings started to rear their ugly heads again now the actual alcohol was out of my body.

I hadn't thought of adding up the cost of the booze that I'd consumed over the years until now. I started drinking in my mid-teens, was now 47, so more than thirty years. God, my poor body and wallet. I had drunk my way through a horrendous amount of money; I was too ashamed to even write the full extent of it down. It was disgusting. But it had stopped! I wanted to spend my money on great, positive things: treats for OH, fun days out, a new coat for the dogs! Maybe even some sensible things, like bills. It was a fresh sunny day and I was alive and getting healthy and that was the most important thing.

The emotional costs ran far higher than the money, without a doubt. At least I was doing something about it. I didn't exactly have my dancing shoes on these past days, but had them on today, and was feeling pretty dapper, despite owning up that I had many thousands outstanding and was trying not to think about it; just a total mess really, but hey, I was alive.

The issue of sugar addiction was starting to bother me – it has always bothered me really but when drinking I could avoid doing anything really serious about it. I had lost about a stone and a half through the diverticular disease getting worse over the last year or so, but I was still about 2 and a half stone over what I wanted to be. I still considered myself relatively fit (I could do a 40-minute run or swim non-stop) but I could go further and faster if I was lighter. I was treating myself with a couple of servings of cake or ice-cream per day, and way too many biscuits and chocolates, simply because my body craved sugar night and day. I didn't expect to lose any more weight as quickly as when I first stopped drinking. But I hoped to again, once I had fully adjusted.

It was around this time that I started to research sugar addiction and consider if the real enemy in my life was not fat, but sugar.

Then came the wedding anniversary. I was more scared of going out this evening than any other time, because I wanted to prove to myself I could do nights out, any kind of night out, especially celebrations, without getting half cut. The restaurant did not have a drinks licence so people were bringing in crates of the stuff. It was like a bottle factory in there. I took a bottle of pretend red wine with me while all around people were gradually getting sloshed, getting lively, getting silly. My alcohol-free sugar syrup tasted rubbish and I felt like cracking. I looked at my husband, who knew from my body language how tricky I was finding it, and I knew I had to stay strong. Just wish I had taken my furry ear muffs as the noise of drunken revellers was most intrusive.

Day 23
Chillaxing (the sun is shining).

Quite a rollercoaster I was on. The last couple of days I had been mostly thinking about anger management, but woke up that morning feeling pretty serene. I guessed all those different emotions were actually what non-drinkers did and dealt with on a regular basis and what I had been avoiding most of my life. Anger was OK – and as so many wise owls pointed out online, was a part of the process of grief – quite a few bereavements of different kinds needed sorting in my head.

We went out for a meal last night, celebrating a friend's wedding anniversary, and surrounded by drinkers. It was a restaurant where you brought your own and there were gallons of the stuff everywhere you looked. People were staggering to the toilets trying to look normal, people getting lairy and loud, supping and supping like their lives depended on it.

Might sound holier than thou but I didn't care … I just felt great knowing I was going to wake up this morning bright and breezy, mentally well, looking forward rather than back. I was terrified I would feel jealous of all those party goers but I just felt smug, unashamedly so, because I had worked hard for this alcohol-free state I was an inhabitant of now and I damn well deserved to be proud of my citizenship. I was also anxious about what the company we were with would say about my non-drinking, but there were no adverse comments and I was actually able to engage better with people than when I gradually got woozy. So that barrier was overcome. Bring it on. Alcohol was just a state of mind.

Day 24
Ridiculous things I did as a drinker.

Stuff I had done on the booze seemed laughable from where I was now sitting, on my little self-proclaimed AF pedestal. I was having a mini smug phase and feeling mildly shamefaced about it, but from a purely selfish point of view, it was helping me stay strong.

I once did this stuff:

- Eating a healthy salad and washing it down with a bottle of wine.
- Going to the gym then going to the pub.
- Pouring the miserable few dregs from my glass back in the bottle because I know I would want it later and could not bear to waste a drop.
- Watching the clock until my self-styled sophisticated, civilised wine o'clock arrived and then glugging a bottle within an hour.
- Pouring a couple of small glasses for me and OH and drinking from the bottle at the same time before taking the delicate little glasses into the living room and sipping it reaaaally slowly, but keeping going back in the kitchen to glug more from the bottle in between refreshing our little glasses.
- Having a preload of wine before going out for a civilised drink with people I knew didn't quaff much and would raise an eyebrow if they saw how I liked to drink.
- Taking the car somewhere under the pretence of not drinking but then having to leave it somewhere because I relented and got drunk instead.
- Buying alcohol presents for people in advance of their birthday but then drinking it instead.
- Searching the house high and low for the places where OH had hidden the drink he didn't want me to have.

Others added to the list:

- Going to the shops for another bottle of wine or more lager/cider, even though there was plenty left, through fear of running out.
- Panicking at the restaurant table if others were drinking at a moderate pace and I needed to get it down me.
- Panicking when dining with friends or family who drank moderately and actually debating in my head if it was bad manners to sip from their glass when they were out of the room, to hurry the drinking the hell up.
- Having reverse beer goggles, where you suddenly decided that after a bottle or two of wine you were completely irresistible to the opposite sex, or even to people of your own sex.
- Ordering a single spirit or small glass of wine when it was someone else's round but doubles or even triples/large glasses when it was your own.
- Having a hair of the dog in the morning and telling yourself it was for medicinal purposes only – more like a full coat once you got going …
- Doing exercise with a hangover just to show how much it didn't affect me, then spending the rest of the day in bed crying and shaking,
- Believing that all of the above was in some way fun, fun, fun
- Dragging slightly bemused friends into my home, so I could say 'Look who's come round! Get the glasses out!'

Day 25

I like girls who drink wine and get out of their minds …

The line of some crappy choon that came on the radio this morning, and it made me think yes, I bet you do, you sad loser, because when a girl is pissed out of her brain you don't have to try so hard …

And then I got to thinking of the power I gave away as a young, vibrant woman, so many times. I allowed myself to be taken over and disrespected by others and by myself. It was a bit of an epiphany because I always considered myself strong, independent, feisty, and so on. The difference was that I was actually being that person, not a version of her diluted by Cabernet.

As women we give away so much when we drink. Things that are precious, priceless even. Stuff we aren't taught to value so much, because we aren't taught that we are important human beings. I thought of alcohol abuse as a feminist issue – all that ladette stuff about keeping up with the men when out drinking was deluded. If I was staggering around paralytic, getting ill, passing on a legacy of self-abuse and addiction to young women who saw me doing it, what on earth was I thinking of? Women have been targeted so aggressively by wine adverts before their favourite television programmes. Alcohol is so bad for girls. It's bad for our boys too but it is a simple scientific fact that women cannot safely process as much wine as men. If you want evidence of this, look at the official guidelines: the NHS recommends no more than 2-3 units a day for women, but 3-4 for men.

I thought what Sarah Turner, co-author of *The Sober Revolution*, talked about in terms of 'mother's little helper' and 'mother's ruin' when I saw her speaking at an event. She discussed how alcohol and drugs have been used historically. That perhaps we are emerging from the wreckage of one of those periods when it seemed acceptable for women to use substances to ‘get by’; in our generation’s case, a bottle of Pinot a night.

It was easy to sweat the small stuff when we consider the issues around getting sober. The withdrawals were bad, but they were doable. The Friday night wobble was pretty rubbish, but I worked through it each week and felt so relieved each new Saturday morning.

Yes, it was boring suddenly having hours free in the evening, or on a lazy Sunday, which used to be filled with boozing. It was problematic deciding what to say or do on nights out where I used to be the first to the bar. These were common threads in most people’s journeys. But there was a much bigger picture too. A political one; where we all play a part if we choose. I wanted to empower myself and achieve things I never dreamed of as a pisshead. I wanted to influence future policy on alcohol by making important buying and lifestyle choices. I wanted to let other women (and men) know that being sober is a lifestyle choice with as much value as any other positive lifestyle choice. Most of all I wanted to show the world that I was strong, my body and mind was my own, and I no longer needed to be out of my mind just to exist, but to enjoy existing. I felt I could start to demand acceptance for who I was.

Day 26
Taking things in hand.

I was in that hiatus period that people seemed to get to after three weeks or so, once the initial challenge had worn off and the new routines started to kick in, and I got that feeling of well, I've proved I can do it, so what now. Well, life was the answer. I do life. The real thing, not the drug induced-haze.

I felt like I was driving myself relentlessly and some days, especially around 6 p.m., it was pretty tricky, but I had found that by repeatedly riding out the fear and the urge to drink, it did pass, and the feeling got shorter the more often I stood up to it. I could not say I was safe yet, as I was acutely aware that the drink could sneak up on people when they were either at their most vulnerable or complacent. If it wasn't for the online blogs by people doing it too, I would not have got this far.

Writing continued to be reassuring and confirming. I felt I was part of a movement for change and my actions were somehow symbolic of how strong women can be when they put their mind to it, and the ones who need a little extra support should get it in spades, no matter how many times they ask for it. I also found I was actually enjoying recording that I was not drinking more than I thought possible. Especially the daily experience of waking up with no regrets and full of optimism. The best thing of all was seeing how happy my hubby was to have his wife present in the moment. I just hoped I could continue like that, knowing it could sneak up on me, and I was very aware that I was still cocooning myself from tricky social situations.

I definitely had wobbles, but was still going.

Day 27
Alcohol get stuffed.

I kept having to pinch myself that tomorrow would be the end of my fourth week off the drug alcohol. With the physical symptoms subsiding, I felt I could start turning my attention to real life and other issues that needed dealing with.

At work two observations had been booked in for me next month and my first thought was, oh I better not have a drink the night before those days as I need to be on top form, then it hit me – not a problem, man! Get in!

Simple pleasures rediscovered or discovered for the first time. It was lovely when that happened; that little flutter of excitement at the discovery of a new way of thinking about what would have been a problem event. It was still so easy to forget I was now a non-drinker and act like a drinker with all the complicated organising and disguising that used to go with it, but what a grand feeling when I reminded myself that nothing was a problem any more because being half cut just didn't have to put in the equation first.

I hoped I wasn't destined to always feel so isolated and did have genuine moments of feeling lonely when it seemed like all the world was drinking and handling it except me and a few unfortunate others. I liked to think in my stronger days that being sober made me enlightened. I hoped that in 10 years' time far more people would be AF.

Day 28
4 weeks down and chucking out some old rules.

It was time for a clear out, and thinking of how I would celebrate this four-week milestone. I had never really considered getting this far but it got easier and easier as the old me got left further behind. Each time I considered going back to old ways, I thought about what I had achieved and how alcohol could never give me this feeling of pride.

So the rules which were redundant were:

- Don't drink in the morning because that means I am an alcoholic.
- Don't drink before 5 p.m. because that means I'm an alcoholic.
- Don't drink every day because that means I'm an alcoholic.
- It's OK to down the first glass in one as long as I sip the second.
- It's OK to finish the bottle because it's silly putting a little snifter back in the fridge.
- It's OK to have 3 cans of cider if wine has made me feel ill.
- It's OK to drink from the bottle in other people's houses as long as I am in the kitchen and they don't see.
- It's OK to keep a ready supply of Tramadol for hangovers but tell the doctor it's for back pain.
- It's OK to have the odd day off work because my body and mind have packed in due to a hangover.
- It's OK to be taken home early from a night out because I had so big a preload I am drunk before I even go out.
- It's OK to cry when I look at my bloated body and know I am going to be fat and unfit forever, because drink is more important than my physical health.

Daftness in the extreme, but there was a time when I still believed I could do moderating as long as I followed rules like those. Now I loved my life and would never go back to that shallow and superficial pissed-ness of life before being AF.

I thanked the 'Drink Demon' for leaving me to my own devices more often these days. There was a time when the little devil would be with me everywhere. There were a few places where it wouldn't be seen dead, incidentally. Like the hospital for a broken ankle (dodgy things those stacked heels, especially with half a litre of vodka on board), or the RTA its victim drove into, the cop shop for a DUI, or the divorce lawyer's office after a drunken affair, or the shrink's office for pills and drink overdose, or in front of a magistrate/judge for neglecting the kids, or any of the other places where it will leave its victim to rot because they have just gone too far this time. After all, once the Drink Demon was bored with you, there were plenty more out there to have fun with.

Day 29
Cravings needed to go.

I had a driving ambition for as much sugar and general crappy food as I could possibly get away with in a day since going AF, and although it had fallen away a bit, it was still giving me cause for concern.

Today I woke up after a solid 7.5 hours (0.5 very important after recently getting a maximum of 5 hours a night) knowing that I actually didn't want a whole packet of custard creams for breakfast and that a packet (or two) of salt and vinegar crisps would not be a reasonable second course. I thought about making my own soup and whereas a few days ago I would have thought soup, yuk, that morning I was thinking what a brilliant idea, get some proper nutrients and make this old body strong again.

I lost 10 pounds in the first three weeks without trying, but it had come to a standstill and so I was going to make the best of this side effect of going AF and carry on losing a few more, but not with biscuits/cookies and crisps, but with some proper healthy meals and a healthier perspective. The question was what would work for me, because I was damn sure I wouldn't stick to a diet. I had 'tried' every diet going and never been able to keep them up, felt bored and frustrated above all hungry and deprived by them. I had to find a way of eating that suited me, gave me freedom to be flexible but was good for my body. Diets always felt so temporary and artificial – I wanted a way of eating for life.

Day 30
Where did all this fear come from?

Up and down on this funny little trundling rollercoaster. I had been awake pretty much all night, dealing with a sudden onset of memories, stuff I hadn't considered for years or ever, trying to get to the bottom of where all this fear came from that generated such compulsive drinking. I spent my entire life being scared of what might happen and trying to offset it, but I could not for the life of me put my finger on what exactly I had been afraid of.

I didn't drink much at all until the last year of sixth form, before that having spent all my time outdoors with horses and friends, and very rarely in the house. I had a steady boyfriend who was unfaithful then finished with me when I was 18 after three years, leaving me bereft. I started going out at weekends with new friends I picked up to stop feeling alone, rather than because we had anything in common, and the habit of Friday and Saturday night pissedness began. This was followed by mid-week drinking added on as the weekend partying was no longer enough.

This getting pissed three to four times a week lasted for a further 30 years, gradually expanding until I drank pretty much every day, congratulating myself if I managed a day off, but always the expectation was that I would enjoy drinking even more after one.

I got myself an interview with a local paper for a trainee reporter job, but drank two double gins before the interview and messed it up. I will never forget the look on the personnel officer's face, my loyal sponsor, in the lift after the interview, knowing I was smelling of gin and had effed up my chance. Aged 17.

At 18, I was told I had to go to university. It was foul. I was lonely, skint because I drank all my grant, so I got a job in a pub in the evenings (naturally) and went clubbing after closing time, and scraped a third in a course I hated from the word go. Got into a lot of debt, solidified my drinking habit, felt abandoned and lonely, always lonely, even in a crowd. My beloved horse-riding and writing were barely evident. Partying was everything. I lost my self-esteem in a series of unsuitable rendezvous with strangers and then drank some more to block out the grieving.

Straight into jobs I hated to solve the debt problem, working in fundraising and public relations, where drinking and long hours were normal and in fact socialising with clients/sponsors was expected. All this time I never made the link between my money, loneliness problems, and my drinking. Met a guy who drank and partied more than me, frequently ending up in a bush on the way home because he couldn't put one drunken foot in front of the other, regularly wet the bed, and later on I found out he was seen in town wrapped round other women. I stayed with him for 5 years, put up with his antics, got engaged because I was desperate to try and rework the relationship. He bought me a £30 ring and three months later called it off. Still scared of being alone, I broke up and made up with him several times, before he met someone else and didn't tell me he had proposed to her, and I found out when one of my friends accidentally witnessed his stag do. How deluded and naive I was. But more partying made it go away.

Binned off the fundraising/PR and went back to uni to train to be a teacher, which I have done ever since with a couple of breaks where depression got the better of me and I needed a break, and teaching had to a large extent both damaged and saved me. If I could not be a professional writer I could at least teach. The half-done manuscripts sat there, taunting me, daring me to finish them.

In 1993 I met my first husband in a night club, naturally, as I spend most of my time in them; I was drunk, of course. In my mid-twenties, as I was then, if I wasn't at work, I was either drinking or recovering from drinking, or getting ready to start drinking. He was charming, 7 years older, the complete opposite of my last rogue of a (younger) boyfriend, a career policeman with money and a house and cars and 'stuff'. For a girl in debt and with no roots to speak of, plus creeping loneliness, even when surrounded by people, he presented himself as an attractive catch.

I saw off his poor little dumpy girlfriend and moved myself in. The violence started soon after, first with a split lip after a row, then a kick in the shin, then a sprained back, and bruises, but never on the face. He drank, I drank, we split up; he charmed me back, we drank, it was violent. Over and over. No room for children in that crazy life. I got my horse, my four-wheel drive, my superficial, materially comfortable existence at the expense of my sanity. What a price to pay. What a dumbass.

There followed weekend dinner parties and on-the-surface civilised behaviour. We got married, of all things. Why did I do that? What was I scared of that was worse than his fists, his venom, his spit in my face, his sly emotional and verbal torture, his strange Other Life that kept him away from the house but which he refused to explain, his impotency with me and yet his extensive porn collection pushed in my face, and his financial secretiveness? What could have been worse than sleeping alone in that marital home, for years, crying and talking to myself in the mirror when pissed, leaving him and then making a fool of myself in my second home, local nightclubs, grieving for my promised fantasy, going back because I was idiotic enough to believe the charm and the promises and the 'let's start again and I promise it will be different' gifts?

What could have been worse than his own mother seeing him strike me to the ground on one of those promised holidays, following a row about chopping up firewood of all things, and for her to pretend nothing had happened? What could be worse than me threaten to report him to his police employers and have a threatening phone call from some stranger promising what would happen to me if I dared 'take the matter further'? What could be worse than spending close to a decade hoping, believing, that something would change for the better that next year, if only I did as I was told and changed too? What could be worse than not having children in my child-bearing years because I truly believed they would be in danger? I later found out this person, this man that I actually married, was investigated after one of his many girlfriends made a complaint about him supposedly exposing himself to her six-year-old daughter.

I had never been able to be alone. I have never been able to ditch the drink because I would lose my most loyal friend and be truly alone. Drink was always the common denominator. I was smashed throughout my wedding day – there was a picture up in a local boozer of me leaning on a beautiful marble fireplace with my hired, badly fitting wedding dress on, a cigarette in one hand and a pint of cider in the other, looking completely vacant. The picture amused many of the punters.

Eight or so years later and crying at work, tears dripping on the morning register and a little girl trying to cheer me up by saying, 'your hair looks nice today, miss'. Didn't know where I was or what I was doing, slowly cracking up, and drink on my breath after another six in the morning row and slap. The tickle never happened.

The head sent me home and told me not to come back until 'whatever it was' was sorted out. I packed a couple of co-op carrier bags and went to an acquaintance's, a girl who had shown me a little kindness one day, who kept her horse at the same livery yard as mine. She took me in, gave me a bed, and gave me time. There are angels out there.

Once the summer holidays arrived I went to my brother in America for a month or so and lay in bed or on the beach, still drinking of course, not much company for him at all, and when I got back my lovely friend had found me a farm cottage to rent with space for my horse, and she brought hers there too. It wasn't until I caught her stealing diesel from the farmer's tank that I realised she had her own agenda too.

That cottage and that farming community were amazing for the eighteen months I was there. Work gave me leave to sort my head out. I stayed off drink for 6 solid months, never went out except to ride my beautiful Irish mare in the Northumbrian hills. I started to get straight. I wondered if I had had some kind of breakdown while I was married, but I had managed to pull out of it.

I went back to work in September 2001 and worked my socks off, getting glowing reports from OFSTED and my department even got a mention in the local newspaper. I got divorced in 2002 with barely a penny, but didn't care, I had escaped and was alive. For the first time since I could remember I had no partner but I was doing OK and felt alone but not lonely. I was growing up.

But, the Drink Demon crept up on me again, and although I was less socially unsettled in my thirties – the drink was just as frequent but done in the house, privately. We all did wine in the house, lots of it. Horsey social events in the area were always loaded with alcohol. Many did vodka and whisky, but I could never handle it – couldn't handle the wine either, but I kidded myself I could!

I had five years alone after the marriage. I grieved for what I believed I had lost. I mixed with a series of unsuitable internet charmers and players, one of which managed to half-inch my car after I signed it over to him in the dumb, drunken belief that he could fix it for me more cheaply if he had the papers … I know. Another conned a hundred out of me to get a tattoo, that I never got back … I was so lonely and vulnerable, and the vats of red wine never stopped being emptied. Another started stalking me so I had to call the police (reluctantly as I wanted nothing to do with them) and lo and behold the police officer investigating started pestering me sexually too. I seemed to have 'lonely and desperate female mug' written in big black marker pen across my forehead. I became quite hard faced and spent a lot of time with different groups of drinking buddies, and we all managed to convince each other that we were invincible, but really we were ageing drunks, starting to lose our looks and brain cells to drink and panicking accordingly.

When I met the love of my life I was becoming immune to any feelings whatsoever. I had recently had a horrific riding accident (drinking the night before and still pissed) which left me with a short right leg held together with a long pin and nails; an accident which finished my nerve, and I sold my beautiful horse.

I had stopped writing and rarely read a book or watched a film right through, unable to concentrate on anything, functioning at work until a series of bullying incidents and a physical assault by a pupil sent me into another spiral of lonely depression, and yet more time off work. Needless to say I spent more time drinking, now during the day, but I forced myself to wait until midday onwards. My only true friend the Drink Demon was always there to lend a helping hand with rules and justifications.

On my return to teaching, I changed to adult learning and found peace again, but the Drink Demon had a hold of me then and wouldn't let go. In 2007, my husband came into all this and saved my life.

A further seven years on and here I was. Sober, reflective, not so scared. Why? I am loved. Also, I realise the Drink Demon caused the fear. Of course I have had some shit happen, don't we all? I have had plenty of chances to turn lemons into lemonade but I chose to stick my lemons in a glass with some tonic. I just could not, could not, go on like that any more. It would have killed me, certainly mentally, if not physically.

The way I looked at it was I had 30 years of drinking. If I was blessed I could have another 30 years on this planet, not drinking and not being scared. I was halfway through my adult life and this was the time to start actually living. I could be strong. And nothing bad would happen as a result.

That was better.

I felt pretty tranquil after letting all that stuff out; it was weird reading it back, made it real, and I just sighed with relief. I recommend doing it. I was terrified about writing down my story, even that edited version, but it really did wonders for my inner peace, felt quite amazing actually and the obsessive thoughts about alcohol, proper OCD stuff, waned so that there were whole hours where the thought of a drink didn't enter my head.

I was no longer making myself sit down and count days, and seemed to be losing count unless I counted back, or checked religiously in my journal. I reckoned this transition from obsessive to slightly less obsessive counting was healthy, such a turnaround from past weeks where all I was thinking about was how many days I had done.

I realised I was actually crying real tears, properly, soberly, and for so much more than I could understand. I experienced grief for lost opportunities, but this time, it was the next stage on from the raw and present horror of it all.

How many of us would do things differently, if we had the benefit of hindsight? Many people have asked me why I stayed with a man (men) who treated me so badly and I just didn't have an answer, other than I got beaten down so much mentally that I actually believed I would never meet anyone really nice and being with someone was better than being with no one. Life was very different for me since meeting my wonderful husband, and although I regretted not having children, I was glad I didn't subject children to my very unsettled life as it was.

I felt like I was reborn with a fresh burst of self-esteem and strength to continue this journey. I had been hanging on to AF counting of days for grim death and been fiercely protective of my total but then I thought, stop counting days and just keep a rough idea of weeks, and ideally this would slide into months, then years. But then again, I needed to keep going until I got to 100. No reason, other than it was a nice round number.

Every single detail of the past, in addition to what happened above, was too painful for me to explore then, and I could only deal with each day one at a time and get through each one. I reckoned what I had experienced had made me who I was and I hoped I was a capable and intelligent woman. I hope I had empathy and insight because of my experiences and that they were part of my growing strength. It was never too late to try my hand at what I really wanted to do. No need to be afraid any more.

I hoped I was doing a grand job of following my own path.

I had learned from longer-sober people before me, and was part of my recovery that I passed it on, gave it away in order to keep it … on a journey called life, keeping an on-going inventory of my thinking and behaviour, checking constantly for anything that might lead back to my old ways.

I thought long and hard about what I had to do to ensure a safe and happy future, having really felt all the emotions that came with remembering the past. I had to try and let the pain go and consequently heal mentally. It was impossible to forget everything, but each time a memory came to the fore now I could acknowledge it and let it float by, because I had dealt with it already … no more mental somersaults and grieving for 'if' required any more. I knew instinctively my honesty and openness with myself was helping me to get well and received a lot of welcome support from my blogging friends online.

It was always going to be very difficult for me to transition from being a drink-repressed 'child' to an emotionally mature adult when I had spent so much time feeling lost and lonely. Good decisions never seemed to present themselves except with the benefit of 20/20 hindsight, especially if you were essentially loving and trusting. That sneaky Drink Demon seemed to know just when to take advantage of our vulnerability and it had certainly had a field day with me.

It was like a bursting a boil in a particularly difficult place to get at (TMI ha-ha) … The past was hellish but I had to also accept I always had choices and I went down other roads of my own volition; but I could not spend the rest of my life grieving for poor decisions and kicking my own head in for it, which was tricky at the best of times. There were only so many somersaults you could do before you broke a rib. I had to forgive myself, even if forgiving others was still a little tricky.

I could feel myself healing through personal forgiveness and moving on. I saw it as a continuation of my journey of self-discovery, by taking a careful and in-depth look at myself, particularly my behaviours, attitudes and the experiences that contributed to my compulsive and reckless actions over the years. It was quite overwhelming; feelings of guilt, shame, confusion and hurt in abandon. I could hardly bear the thought of reviewing my past in any more detail; it was too painful to think about how I had hurt others and myself and like many before me I questioned the value of opening old wounds. Wouldn't it be better to forget the past entirely and move on? But remembering gave me more insight into who I really was and I knew that the more insight I had, the less likely I was to go back to my old ways.

However hard it was, I had no excuse for the extent of my drinking and in the end no real back story compared to the terrible tragedies suffered by some, except a few decades of feeling just not quite good enough, whatever it was I was doing, and suffering intense anxiety about not doing 'it' right.

Looking back I know I have always had issues, even as a child. I played truant and drank from my parents drink's cabinet secretly during the day because I never fitted in school, was bullied psychologically, although when the school reported my behaviour to my mother, her reaction was to tell me what a disappointment I was, and I have had that comment in my brain ever since.

One of the reasons I became a teacher was to expunge my own memories of school. Once such thing was playing the lead in *Mother Courage* and the head of the English department suggesting I came to his office for extra guidance on playing the role, then proceeding to sit beside me and rub his ugly, hairy hand up and down my leg. I was 14 years old and had no idea what was going on; I thought he was trying to be friendly. A couple of weeks later he and his girlfriend, also an English teacher there, gave me a lift home after a late rehearsal and tried to get me to go in their house, but my common sense prevailed.

When I moved from middle to high school, for some reason they put me in one stream and all my dear horsey friends in another stream, and I was completely isolated with a load of chav bullies who made it their business to rip the piss on a daily basis. I remember one of them saying, 'Is it raining outside?' and I innocently answered no, thinking it was an ordinary question and for once she was being approachable, then they all howled because really they were taking the piss out of my greasy hair. I could go on. I am with you if you ever suffered abuse in school.

I grew up with depression, later in my late teens/early twenties with self-harming with self-destructive behaviour such as stupid, pointless shoplifting and thieving, selling my body for the price of a meal and a drink or five and people-pleasing in both professional and domestic situations, which all enabled the Drink Demon to get its hooks deeper in me.

Anyway, I got grown-up physically if not mentally, and gained the insight to start dealing with this (albeit very slowly). Forgiveness? I couldn't forgive myself then, never mind anyone else. How could I forgive the fact that at Uni I was on the night bus after a session and even though I had a widdle before getting on the bus I was so desperate I knew I would wet my pants if I didn't get some relief, so, full of drink, I slipped off my jeans to my knees and weed into the seat at the back of the bus, What I didn't realise was that it would drip onto the floor and make a puddle round my feet and I also didn't realise that I was in direct view of the mirror thing the driver uses to spy on people on the top deck. What a look I got from him when I did the walk of shame off that vehicle.

Another shameful episode was having to stop at a friend's house because I was too pissed to find a taxi and get home on my own, so she insisted I stayed with her, bless her for keeping me safe. I fell unconscious as soon as she heaved my semi-conscious carcass diagonally onto the bed (I am six foot so that takes some doing) but woke up in the middle of the night feeling both rough and sodden everywhere because I had wet myself. That poor girl who had looked after me and kept me safe then had to deal with a load of piss-soaked bedding, me in hysterical tears of shame crowning a Grade A hangover, and a ruined mattress. It took me back to a day when I was maybe six or seven, and a group of older girls took me to a distant field and made my take my clothes off and wee in front of them, before leaving me to get dressed and find my own way home, laughing their heads off. I was shouted at and given the slipper on my bare behind when I finally got home, because I was late for tea.

I offered to pay for the bedding and mattress but she refused, and I guess she just wanted this vile cavewoman out of her house. I wasn't invited out by that group again.

A few years later and when I got divorced I spent a few months looking at houses to buy, I had had a heavy session the night before I went to see this particular house, and was caught with severe tummy problems in the middle of the viewing (thankfully I was alone). I tried and failed to get up to the toilet and just managed to get my kegs off before World War 3 happened all over the living room floor. Thankfully it was a bare wood floor, but I was then presented with the logistics of removing diarrhoea from the floor boards of an empty house, plus as they had my details they would know it was me that did it, and what if someone was viewing after me … they would be presented with a huge pile of biology. So I went out in the back yard in a panic looking for any kind of implement, nothing around except a soaking wet pile of old newspapers, so I had to make the best of a bad job, practically howking my guts up the whole time with the smell and the general savagery of it. What a dirty dog.

Onwards and upwards. The past was gone. The now and the future was all there was.

Husband took me out for lunch after he read this entry this morning, and we both got upset and got angry about some of it; he didn't know any of that stuff, so we talked it out. Poor lad, learning what his beloved was really like.

A wonderful friend read my story and told me her feelings about what happened in her past: 'Despite all my crying, I was nonetheless proud and surprised by the strength I felt I demonstrated, in order to combat my drinking, as well as the realisation that the alcohol was causing my fear. My fear was certainly intense and because I smoked too, I had double fear! My fear lifted when I got sober and I felt able to leave the paralysis behind me. I watched a documentary about OCD recently and the children all feared horrible things happening to their loved ones if they didn't ritualise when they had 'the thoughts'. The leaders drew question marks on the kids' wrists so they had a visual to look at when they had the negative thoughts. The question marks signified, 'maybe something bad will happen or maybe it won't' and I have tried to turn my thinking to that. I refuse to keep catastrophising every pain or twinge I have, deeming it to be something awful as a result of my drinking. Crying, crying, crying, and feeling calm. A total release. I am not underestimating the significance of my tears and the intensity of how I feel. I hope I can share and help some people. Increasingly, I want to do something concrete to help others going through the same stuff, even with different life scenarios. I want people to know they are not alone and never will be, as long as they are honest and reach out. Denial was only going to cause heartache. I have decided to enjoy the next 30 years, giggling, loving, being loved, living, being.'

Day 31
Recognise yourself? I did when I read this.

Courtesy of the NHS website in the UK. Thank you NHS for all the work you do to help drinkers and victims of drinkers.

Obsessive compulsive disorder (OCD) is a mental health condition where a person has obsessive thoughts and compulsive behaviour. An obsession is an unwanted, unpleasant thought, image, or urge that repeatedly enters a person's mind, causing them anxiety. The word 'obsession' usually describes something enjoyable, but in OCD the obsession is unpleasant and frightening.

A compulsion is a repetitive behaviour or mental act that someone feels they need to carry out to try to prevent an obsession coming true. For example, someone who is obsessively scared they will catch a disease may feel the need to have a shower every time they use a toilet.

OCD symptoms

OCD symptoms can range from mild to severe. For example, some people with OCD may spend an hour or so a day engaged in obsessive-compulsive thinking and behaviour. For others, the condition can completely take over their life. Although OCD affects individuals differently, most people with the condition fall into a set pattern of thought and behaviour. The pattern has four main steps:

- Obsession – your mind is overwhelmed by a constant obsessive fear or concern, such as the fear your house will be burgled.
- Anxiety – this obsession provokes a feeling of intense anxiety and distress.
- Compulsion – you adopt a pattern of compulsive behaviour to reduce your anxiety and distress, such as

checking all your windows and doors are locked at least three times before leaving the house.

• Temporary Relief – the compulsive behaviour brings temporary relief from anxiety but the obsession and anxiety soon return, causing the cycle to begin again.

Some elements of OCD in its entirety didn't fit for me but I thought the routines that as a drinker I needed to follow to feel safe were part of an obsessive-compulsive syndrome of some sort, may be not severe enough to be hospitalised, but enough to interfere with me making a success of my life, and certainly causing a good deal of depression, stress, and anxiety.

Day 32
Obsessions that didn't matter any more.

At work today, I interviewed a gentleman in his fifties and was knocked sideways by the alcohol on his breath. The whole room stank of it. I was shocked that he felt able to come in in that state, but I was ashamed to admit I was also fascinated that someone so completely unaware of their problem could be carrying on life as if nothing was the matter. He appeared perfectly sane and normal and had it not been for the whiff, I would never have guessed he was in the middle of his own private hell.

It took me back, as so many things did at that moment, to a time in the middle of my first marriage, when I was parish clerk for a couple of years in the little village we inhabited, and the fact that I always went to the meetings with wine on my breath after my dinner, and maybe people knew. They certainly knew after I went to see the chairman to hand my notice in one morning at 10 a.m., to his lovely home, his private space, with a few glasses of whisky in me because my lovely ex-husband had spat on me on his way to work, ending a row which had been bubbling like a cauldron for days. I couldn't pretend to be normal any more and was starting to withdraw from everyone.

I was naive to assume no one in the village knew of my traumas and my drinking. Our rows would have carried to the far end of the green. I remember a lady with a greyhound picking me off the ground one evening. I had wandered out into the lane after more rowing and him pushing me to one side outside the bathroom, slamming the door with my foot jammed under it, so I fell and twisted both my ankle and my back. I was just sitting there on the tarmac in my drunken stupor, in pain, not knowing where I was and actually rather hoping a tractor might run me over and take the decision to finish my existence out of my hands. She tried to get me to go home with her, this stranger, but I refused. I went to the pub instead and blagged drinks off the landlady, and slept on her sofa overnight. My husband didn't come looking for me.

It was pretty exhausting to write this stuff, but tiring in the same way as I might have felt after a good day out with someone I cared about, and was wrung out emotionally but knew something good had happened. This process of blood-letting was 'the norm' for addicts in recovery, I read, and this was actually what happened when people were on the road to wellbeing. No doubt I would have bursts of other stuff to remove from my psyche. I just hoped people who read it realised it was not a call for help as such; it was a cathartic process that was actually making me better and that if they were in mental pain and could think of doing it too, they could experience a big shift in their stores of strength.

Day 33
Am I happy or am I just nuts?

I was upset first thing today and getting tearful and I actually gave myself a hug and told myself how well I was doing. It wasn't planned, the pep talk just happened. It felt bloody good and I cheered myself right up instead of telling myself off, for a change.

I kept getting rushes of a sense of liberation and a knowledge that the world was opening up ahead of me, cocking a finger and saying, do you dare find out who you really are and what you are capable of?

I could not work out in my mind if this was causing me happiness or if I was actually round the bend, simply because I didn't think I had ever experienced true happiness, not deep down. I was not sure what to do with this feeling.

I always put a cap on happiness because that would mean that a) I am ergo not concerning myself with what other people needed for their happiness if I was thinking about my own and b) I didn't feel I had a right to it in any circumstances and should maintain a constant state of anxiety. I was a disappointment to certain people and have always felt that I was letting people down; never quite being good enough in other's eyes. I just never reached their expectations. Drinking was a great way to a) make myself into someone else and b) to forget that important people in my life didn't rate me too highly, even if they did their best to cover it up. Except my number one man of course, who was everything to me. To have completely unconditional love, to sense no disappointment or have to deal with 'why don't you' statements was completely new.

So I reckoned I might give this happiness thing a go and see what happened. Tentatively. For once, I would try hard not to put a time limit on it.

I was still waiting for my soup maker; my flask had

arrived though so I was half ready for Operation Soup for Lunch. Happiness was all about appreciating what I did have, for instance the metaphorical flask instead of the soup maker and actually allowing myself to be happy, instead of trying to control it all the time like I used to try and control the drinking.

The reasons I drank were complex but I always felt one of the main ones was to blot everything out. Plus a drink instantly started the party atmosphere. Another was to douse anger.

The times I have really been tempted in any of the last few weeks has been in response to anger. I have managed to keep going but it has made me aware that I was suddenly really feeling the emotions and also taking responsibility for myself. It was me that made me drink and no one else. Why not give happiness, or whatever it was, a chance?

Maybe I was not nuts, but a bit scared to be happy. The Drink Demon had robbed me of my self-esteem, so when I became AF and I started to become happier, calmer and more peaceful, it was almost a physical shock.

How heart-warming to know that I could be happy. Most people didn't experience happiness – they just plodded on without questioning their state of mind. Self-awareness made me a lucky one. I was experiencing that fantastic feeling of freedom that comes with knowing myself better and it felt bloody good. I had never felt or been told I was good enough, but I learnt to love myself a bit more since giving up drinking.

Day 34
When is a routine not a routine?

When it becomes a compulsion. I managed to drop a few drink-related 'compulsions' which I used to think of as my safe little routines, but actually they were things I clung to because stopping them would be too risky.

All around me I saw drinkers with obsessions and compulsions which they considered normal … after having read that book *Why Be Happy When You Can Be Normal?* – well for drinkers 'normal' is something that when you look back on it makes your flesh creep.

Routines:

- Having a must-have type of glass for certain drinks or else it wouldn't taste right – no wine in a mug, bejesus.
- Having to have certain drinks made and served in a certain way or they wouldn't be successful drinks (ice and lemon with that?).
- Having to have the glass filled to a certain level or it was unsettling, that is if it got too full or too short a measure (can you top that up for me please?).
- Doing the same number of sips/glugs at certain points, sip the top off, glug a bit, sip a bit so not to seem rude, wait till someone else has finished theirs before gratefully finishing it and waiting for a refill.
- Never allowing anyone to get to the situation of a completely empty glass (esp. my glass) or the world would end.
- Matching my company's drinking so I didn't miss out on or end up getting an extra round, as that would mean I was out of kilter and uncomfortable, not one of the 'guys'.
- Drinking wines that I felt suited my mood (don't feel like red tonight, let's have a cheeky rosé, or a bit of

fizz, darling).

- Having certain drinks at certain times of day (spirits this early, my dear what a *faux pas*).

God.

I decided I could allow myself the habit of nice drinking vessels for my new AF compulsion, which after all was not going to kill me or break up relationships and so on.

I had a proper AF date last night with my OH. We went out in the pissing rain and wind and walked along the beach in the dark, not a soul there, watching the fireworks in the sky, holding hands, getting blown all over. The waves were crashing and the seagulls were circling. We went and sat in a cafe and had freshly cooked fish and chips and then handed over a tenner in an amusement arcade. I gave my winning tokens to a little girl who was standing by the prize stall looking wistful, and I felt really good because it wasn't a drunken gesture, it was real, and the smile on her mother's face wasn't apprehension because I was lairy, it was genuine surprise and delight. This morning I remembered every single part of our date and I felt about twenty years younger. That experience was for me the true essence of the main thing.

Day 35
Confessions of a biscuit eater.

I was not having any urges for alcohol at all as the end of five weeks approached; in fact the thought of it just sickened me. I felt like I had made a positive choice and was proud to be part of a group of people online who had worked so hard to make a difference to their lives and wellbeing. This included people who were still struggling – the fact was that they had decided to do something about it, no matter how long it took, and that was something to be really proud of. I hoped they would not give up.

The problem I had was that I had replaced compulsive drinking with compulsive sugar eating. I had never really bothered with biscuits before, but I was eating the same weight in Fox's as I used to do in Hardys and Magners before. Last night I stuffed half a treacle tart down me before bed and this morning demolished the other half before 7 a.m. as it was burning a hole in my brain, just knowing it was there. I was now a size 12 from a 16, and had lost 4 inches off my bra size, but I had a feeling if this sugar thing continued I would undo the good work. Sugar made me feel ill and mentally not right in a similar way to alcohol and I decided that I was going to tackle this in the same way I did the drink. It was going to be interesting finding out what my addictive brain replaced sugar with.

I had been battling headaches for a while and it never once crossed my mind that they could be sugar-related, until I started researching the effect that sugar had on our bodies and then it became obvious that pretty much all my continuing 'morning hangover' symptoms were not alcohol but sugar related.

As I was feeling safe in my sobriety now it was well worth cutting out the extras, and I was sure I would get some energy back as a result.

At the same time I had to begrudgingly say thank you to the sugar; it had done its job well in helping me get sober and now I was in a safe place to get rid of it.

I wanted to keep small amounts of fruit and natural unprocessed sugar, but the added extra pure refined stuff (sounds posh, 'refined', but clearly not) had to go. Experts told me that my blood sugar would stabilise then, pootling along at normal healthy levels, no highs and lows that made me feel odd and wanting more, more, more.

I thought it was also a good idea to focus on the good stuff as well as letting out the bad.

Good things this week:

My soup maker was on its way. I had veggies growing in the garden which would make lovely soups for lunch. My flask was new and shiny and waiting. The soup maker also did smoothies. I was excited about this gadget in a way I never would have been when a bottle was all that I looked forward to.

The biscuit craving was getting on my nerves now instead of saving me, so I was doing a lot of mental preparation for getting rid of this habit. I planned my food in advance today and would be 'using' fruit when the biscuit urge struck – no doubt I would have to deal with fruit obsession at some point but one step at a time.

I bought a sketch pad and a little tray of water colours. So the 100 odd programmes I recorded off the Painting and Drawing Channel (OCD) can start to be watched with a little brush in hand. It was nuts, especially bearing in mind the results, but it was better than drinking. Everything was better than drinking.

I managed to ride the panic and drink-wobbles enough times in recent weeks to know the craving passed if you gave it space. It just meant developing a coping mechanism involving thinking through step by step what would happen after you took that first drink. Made yourself follow through as it were, so that you imagined the way you would feel after a bottle and how disappointed you would be in yourself. It was just not worth taking that first drink. Write the process down and by the time you have written your little flow chart, the urge will have passed, drinking will seem utterly pointless, and you will feel stronger for your decision.

Day 36
Happy Birthday, me, and 10 things that have replaced alcohol.

I counted my blessings as I headed into Week 6. I tried to decide I was not fussed about counting as I felt this was my permanent way of life now, but it was all the same human nature to think about milestones and be proud of stuff achieved based on time measures. So I would still count away if it got me there; everyone could go AF, no matter what method they favoured.

While I was in a counting mood I was thinking of all the stuff I had replaced alcohol with:

1. I turned the telly off more and read. Before AF (BAF? BARF?) I would sit with a glass and stare at the goggle box for hours, having my brain hoovered by the drink and the telly at the same time. Still watched a load of crap but I was far less tolerant of it. It drove my OH mad when I kept muting things because they did my head in now, whereas before it just washed through my dazed brain. The telly was often off.

2. I took longer walks. One of the ways I dealt with coming off drink in the first days was being away from temptation as much as possible, and it had become a nightly habit now with OH and the two terriers. In the past going for an evening walk would have been rushed through and not enjoyed really, so I could get back to either finish or start the wine/cider/lager.

3. Talking to people online more and making friends. I had spent literally hundreds of hours online. I was on it all the time. I needed it and loved it. I was so grateful for people posting blogs and commenting on my blogs so I could read their stuff, and felt stronger when people took time to talk to me. I was unashamedly needy of other AF people at that moment. I felt unsettled and uncomfortable when people talked about moderation, but that was

something in me I needed to deal with.

4. I was getting honest to God, straight-up feelings. When I stopped stopping life, a lot of really unsettling feelings started to happen in my head, but they were also exciting. I felt like I was observing some sort of scientific experiment happening in my brain. I didn't know where my anger and crazy eureka moments would take me but it was going to be interesting finding out and for the first time I did actually want to find out, not stop it all in its tracks.

5. I was spending more time looking at and looking after myself. My conditioned self said it was vain and self-indulgent doing all this introspection, and even giving up drinking was a way of trying to be unnecessarily different to everyone else. I should just go with the flow. Actually I liked the fact that my skin was smoother and my face was less bloated and I may be losing some of that leg cellulite.

6. I was being nicer to people. I was ashamed to say I had been a gossip and indiscreet when a drunk, or when bad tempered/moody/hungover, but AF had a way of making me feel more serene and more *laissez faire* generally. People said stuff now and I didn't waste time getting involved, I just let them have their little moan and when they saw I was not jumping in too, they got bored and stopped. I wished I used this strategy years ago and saved myself a lot of awkward and unpleasant situations due to my big mouth.

7. I was spending more time relaxing, mentally and physically. I had replaced the hurry sickness that seemed to accompany drinking and recovering from drinking, where life and people were just so stressy. If I didn't do it today, I would do it tomorrow. It would get done. Sometimes it didn't need doing at all. The world wouldn't end.

8. I was enjoying my work more. I was working harder than ever but actually taking pleasure in it, instead of

struggling through a day wanting to kill people with my bare hands. Spending more time working might not be everyone's cup of tea, but for me being better at my job was replacing a lot of the half-hearted attitudes I had to certain parts of it as a drinker (drink was always more important). Hard work was part of my recovery.

9. I was spending more time thinking about healthy food. The biscuit thing needed to be dealt with and so did chocolate and crisps, but I was enjoying cooking and growing food and thinking about what my body needed instead of what my addiction needed.

10. I was looking forward to the future instead of dreading it. The black cloud seemed to be loitering over there somewhere rather than directly over my head. Nothing in my life was really any different but I was dealing with it differently and that was a priceless feeling.

More counting: it was my birthday today. I was entering my 48th year, but I wouldn't be drowning my sorrows, I would be celebrating the start of a new phase. I actually felt excited.

That night I sat with an AF white wine spritzer with loads of ice, pint glass, burger with onion and cheese, watching Al Pacino in *Insomnia*, with OH. How much further away from alcoholism I could not imagine on a Saturday night and I bloody loved it.

Day 37
Joining the revolution.

Until now I never really thought about my place in the bigger scheme of things, until I read Lucy Rocca and Sarah Turner's *The Sober Revolution* and it made me think about the wider issues, outside of my current bubble. My bossy teacher head was quite tickled by the idea of having a reading list for getting over addiction, like it was that simple; how great that would be if I could study, sit an exam, and then be officially sober. Life, eh?

The book has a lot to say to women about their predicament with drink and some hard truths as well. *The Sober Revolution* discusses the idea of moderation in depth and the fact that IF you have to plan and regulate your drinking, it is not moderating, it is denial. Moderate drinkers don't have to make themselves timetables and focus on resisting drink, nor do they have to justify their actions.

The authors talk about the revolution and how we can all be part of something powerful that can change the world if enough of us join up. Sober, we are all part of a much bigger and more beautiful picture. The thing is, do we want to help paint the picture or be the ones that steal the paint?

The authors talk about being a dry drunk, which I recognised in my life for years and years, congratulating myself on resisting a drink all week and even calling the non-imbibing days AF days, when in fact my body was still full of alcohol and I only resisted as long as the hangover lasted and before the withdrawal set in. It was classic binge drinking, not moderating!

There is also a section on the different types of drinking. Binge drinking, which as I mentioned is resisting for a while and setting parameters for days when you will get blasted – how many hundreds of thousands of people binge drink in this country and how many millions worldwide? That was me in my early twenties. Then there is harmful drinking, which is going over government guidelines – when you think 14 units is the maximum and how much is this in wine terms? A bottle and a half over 7 days! How many of us did that a day? Hazardous drinking by their definition is around a bottle a night. Like maintenance drinking is keeping the levels topped up weekly so you never have a chance to get hungover or for people to notice your whole life is balanced precariously on having both open and secret snifters whenever possible. This 'progresses' to the heavily dependent drinker who most of us think of as the stereotypical alkie, vodka for breakfast and so on.

Also interesting in the book are the stories about women from a wide cross section of society who have experienced drinking problems in all its different guises, including Lucy and Sarah themselves. So much of the detail in these tales is relatively ordinary but more shocking because it is so ordinary – taking the kids to school after drinking the night before and not realising you are double the limit still – getting suspended from work because you ended up in an accident that wasn't your fault but you got breathalysed and got done as a result …

The fact was I didn't need to be having vodka for breakfast to have a really unhealthy addiction to alcohol, and in some ways the lower levels of addiction down from 'heavily dependent' were more deadly because of liver disease not being diagnosed. Often health care professionals simply didn't act unless patients were in the really obvious stages of full-blown alcoholism.

I went to other doctors several times because I was worried about my drinking only to be told, 'Well, cut down then' – oh right, I never thought of that. It was my latest doctor who persuaded me to take an anti-depressant and offered counselling, which I have had to decline because these people only work a 9-5.

Day 38
Making vows.

When I got married to lovely husband number two we wrote our own vows. I meant every one, and I would like to think I have stuck to them. I was thinking of sobriety as a marriage between myself and it, and last night started thinking about the vows I could make to sobriety.

I will not drink. I will look after my body. I will continue to love and cherish my husband. I will write every day. I will find a way to stop feeling guilty about being me. I will stop apologising for being me. I will find a way to love myself.

I thanked my new AF friends online for being there for me unreservedly. Unconditional friendship was very precious. I had never met any of them in the flesh at that point (I did later) but felt very close to them in spirit. I felt much stronger each morning having read their comments.

I had my husband and he had me.

Thanks to a sober friend for telling me: 'it doesn't matter how slowly you go so long as you don't stop.'

I was fed up of feeling negative. I wanted to believe the voice that was telling me that it was selfish/vain to be introspective was not my voice. I told myself I had a right and a duty to myself to give myself some time to actually feel what feels right and wrong for me and to develop and listen to my own authentic voice.

Day 39
The Bright Field.

I was reading a book called *The Mindful Way Through Depression* by John Kabat-Zinn, and though it is not specifically about addiction, a lot of the book called out to people with addictions and encouraged reflection and meditation, in order to find a way through the rumination maze.

I loved this poem by R.S. Thomas quoted in it:

I have seen the sun break through
to illuminate a small field
for a while, and gone my way
and forgotten it. But that was the pearl
of great price, the one field that had
the treasure in it. I realize now
that I must give all that I have
to possess it. Life is not hurrying
off to a receding future, nor hankering after
an imagined past. It is the turning
aside like Moses to the miracle
of the lit bush, to a brightness
that seemed as transitory as your youth
once, but is the eternity that awaits you.

I was thinking about transitions and the in between space on my journey … ever reminding me to be present in the present.

Day 40
What ELSE am I addicted to?

There was a tendency to look back on giving up drink and find it was nowhere near as bad as you'd thought, because now your head was in the right place. It wasn't exactly a walk in the park getting to the point where I had finally had enough, but still. If you knew deep down this was really truly the final curtain for drinking, then going the final step and leaving it behind was actually OK.

I found the slightly scary bit was being left with the stuff that I also did appear to be addicted to, number one of which was of course refined sugar. This battle was proving far harder. It was actually bothering me a lot that I could not go without sweet stuff during the day, and I actually got terrible mental and physical symptoms, like I once did with alcohol, if I didn't have it.

I was still waking up feeling fuzzy. I felt great as the day went on though, which was lovely. I was sure it had to be the sugar – which I had now cut down on, but it obviously took longer to get out of the system.

My reading at this point was *Sugar Blues* by Alan Dufty, who writes eloquently about what sugar does to our insides and our health generally, and how withdrawal affects us. A friend also commented on this excellent book: 'He recommends replacing refined sugar products with sweet juicy fruit and then you introduce more sweet veg to your diet, like pumpkin, sweet potato, to come off gradually. He also recommends veggie juices, for example with raw beetroot, carrot, and ginger which is very sweet.'

I managed no sugar all day today and had a throbbing headache – I was in bed by 7.30 p.m. Research suggested that when beating the sugar and caffeine, headaches subside within 3-5 days.

I realised the protein issue was an important factor in my food choices. I was eating very little protein and all the nutritionists I researched agreed it was so important to ensure protein played a part in each meal.

It was still early days for my 47-year-old body to get used to a new AF life and the sugar cravings would go in time, but only with positive action. During this phase of physical adjustment I had to go with what my body wanted in the knowledge that it would soon be over and biscuit production nationwide could go back to normal. I was determined not to let sugar rule my life like alcohol used to.

Day 41
Head done in.

It would be quite good to have more than one day in a row where my mood was the same. At least with being hungover or even just a little jaded you knew where you were – grumpy and ill. Since I binned the drink, my mind had gone haywire thinking about all the issues that made me drink in the first place and battling with horrendous feelings of guilt about this new-found anger and determination that made me feel good at times, but the fallout wasn't going to have a very positive effect on social life, as I just wanted to be alone.

This didn't go down well when I failed to attend my brother's engagement party, because I had a panic attack about being in a group of people, some of whom I barely knew, without alcohol, when they would all be drinking. I felt weak and pathetic, but apart from us not having a cent to get there, buy even AF drinks or dress up in the first place, I was a wreck in social situations. I could perform at work because I played a set role, but in anything unstructured or unknown, I went to pot. I began to realise my existing dose of anti-depressants were just not working.

I looked into getting some cognitive behavioural therapy training because I thought it was such a fantastic way to heal, and I liked to think I could help others in some way; the classic route of a 're-forming' addict, I guessed. There was a diploma starting at my local university the following autumn, which gave me a year to get my head sorted out and ready to start a new phase.

I lost my rag with a learner today. His jaw dropped really slowly as I let him have it, after his constant whining about having a hangover and being expected to work when all he wanted to do was sleep it off. He stank of stale drink. I felt insulted he would expect my time and support in that state so I told him to get away home. He was astonished as I never shout. Jeez it felt good. He volunteered an apology and gave me double work after that. Bam. Sometimes getting annoyed was OK, as are a lot of feelings we shut out when we drank.

I had to try not to be afraid of these overwhelming emotions – they were scary and shocking too. They were normal though, not drink induced, and sometimes it was good to remember that if I was not feeling like this, then there actually would be something wrong with me. It was the lack of numbness which took some adjusting to.

I was a bit of an emotional mess; one minute I was on top of the world and handing out gems of wisdom to others left right and centre, the next I was a child sitting in the corner with my head in my hands. It was at times like this I wished I was a mum so I could focus on my kids and just love them. Last night I wondered if I was in the middle of some kind of nervous breakdown. However. I was going to the doctor's tonight and hopefully they would sort me out; probably need to up my dose of happy pills.

I tried to remember the only reason anybody could be disappointed in somebody, is because they wanted or expected them or needed them to be somebody they were not, and that was for their own reasons.

Day 42
Six weeks, wobbling, but still there.

I found myself living in a bit of a virtual cyber world; finding the real world was decidedly unattractive.

I was so happy to be celebrating six weeks AF. This week had been my hardest yet because real life and dire memories had got in the way the most, whereas previous weeks I was able to pretty much cosset myself in the flat and keep my mind focused on day to day stuff. The doc doubled my dose of anti-ds and gave me a contact for counselling.

The feelings this strange behaviour of mine created were exhilarating, scary, liberating, and very unusual generally. I had absolutely no idea what would happen next but I would be sober doing it. Sometimes it was good not to know.

I needed to share my feelings about things with others in order to make them real and to stop living with my old low self-worth and self-destructive beliefs. I had got enough sobriety under my belt to know which way I wanted to go and I wanted be able to discover the true me to its finest. If I didn't take care of my emotional wellbeing, who would?

Whether talking online or face to face, it was all real life, just different versions of it with different levels of intrusion. There were certain social groups and situations I found threatening and I thought of them as my 'old' life. What I was doing was laying the foundations for and living a new life; no doubt I would take some elements and people with me and leave others behind. It would just take a while to sort through things.

My reading odyssey continued. Three books about overcoming drink I ordered came today – Tanya Glyde's *Cleaning Up*, Rosie Boycott's memoirs, and Della

Galton's *Ice and a Slice*. I was looking forward to more hours of peaceful reading. Life could be tough at times but it was a whole lot tougher with the booze.

Chapter Three

Releasing more demons

Day 43
Starting week 7 at a crossroads.

I continued to haunt the internet like a non-drinking waif. Reading was pretty much the only thing that kept me going, apart from OH. I mentioned renting him out to help the bills last night. I thought ironing might be a good money spinner; he was good at that.

Having no alcohol on board helped me make the right decisions (probably not including the one about renting out the OH) and gave me freedom to express my preferences.

The booze healed no part of me or my life, all it did was make me repeat the same errors over and over. But I no longer wanted to look back in anger, it was just too exhausting. Sometimes we carried pain and hurt needlessly. We could not change the past and it was OK to be angry about it, but then we needed to leave it behind and move forward. Harrowing and painful though elements of the past may be, I would grow from this. It might not become clear immediately but in a future moment I would reflect, with a sense of calm and peace. For now, I would be gentle on myself and take some time out to sit, and just be.

I felt empowered today and once all the head stuff was cleared up one way or the other I would be a lot calmer. When people treated you badly, either intentionally or through lack of thought, the consequences were their problem; we could only stand up for ourselves in the end and they would have to deal with it.

The lead up to the big AF event involved tears, stress, drama, bullying, and manipulation in order to get me standing there smiling for the camera. My reading and research opened my eyes to some of my own behaviour and how I sometimes didn't listen to what people were trying to tell me because they were not doing what I wanted them to do.

Being AF did bring more clarity and while it was painful I knew it helped me to face my demons.

Day 44
How to look good sober.

I had aired a lot of dirty washing. I had to or I would have drank, simples.

Today I went walking with my partner while the rest of my family and their friends were partying, having all stayed over at their venue last night and staying there again tonight. Tomorrow I would be getting up as normal at 6 a.m. in my slightly dowdy flat, walking my hairy, smelly dogs, and then teaching people who had real poverty and some terrible issues in their lives. Little did my wonderfully demanding and challenging adult learners know how crucially important they had been to me in recent weeks.

I'd been thinking about Gok Wan (I love him) and what he would say to me. Without a doubt it would be, 'Get out there, girlfriend, and love yourself.' I read his autobiography a couple of years ago and he has struggled for years with lack of self-esteem issues around food, but he is such a great example of how to look good no matter what life throws at you. Role models were very important at this point.

I decided to look for other role models and to work on the same things they worked on to get where they were. I had never done that before, but it felt right to try some different routines.

I was conscious of a deep fear of doing anything differently to how I'd always done it, thinking differently, acting differently; it was a true panicky feeling to consider the possibility that things could actually be different if I decided they were. I could choose how I felt and how I reacted, and how much time I spent with people. And there was not a damn thing anyone else could do about it. I would not die, the world would not end, and there would not be some kind of earthquake under my feet or lightning striking me from above. I would just continue. Now that was looking good sober. I decided that the mantra, 'What would Gok say?' was a good one.

Day 45
Things that don't work any more.

Giving up alcohol affected my whole life in ways I had not anticipated. Things that I thought could be dealt with accompanied by a bottle of delightful Prosecco/Chardonnay/Barolo/plonk became pretty much impossible to have in your life once the drug was gone too.

My top ten 'no mores':

1. Certain people. People who drank heavily and smelt of it, people who moaned heavily, people who were bossy and domineering, people who still wanted you to stay in your timid little box.

2. Certain places. Most of my previously haunted bars and pubs, some restaurants where drunkenness happened, some streets in town where shameful things happened.

3. Certain ways of eating. I had a tremendous biscuit craving for weeks and it was doing my nut in, but all of a sudden it was dissipating! Sugary things tasted sugary again rather than just necessary. It was work in progress.

4. Certain routines. I had to change the way and order I did things so normal life didn't continually remind me of times I would need to have a drink. I used to have lazy Saturday afternoons waiting for wine/cider o'clock to strike, but these days I stayed busy. When I got in from work I would have headed straight for the kitchen, but now I had a stretch out on the bed and a cuddle if OH/terriers/all three were around, till the stress went.

5. Certain attitudes. I realised recently that a lot of my life was spent in a permanent state of fear. Fear of what

other people could think, do, say, feel, want from me. Having gone AF I actually felt liberated. I was still here.

6. Certain approaches to life. I have had to make myself positive where before I too easily sank into negative (and drank). My life was not much different from when I was drinking regularly, but I coped better with stress and fatigue because I was no longer either twitchy with a hangover or tense because I had to wait for a drink. Life was life was life; we all had to do it.

7. Drama, crises, and panic stations. I used to act impetuously, madly even, rushing off here and there, always anticipating the worst scenario and trying to remedy it in advance; absolutely crackers and playing right into the hands of alcohol, because that was the only thing that calmed me down. Once after I had been drinking I went into a department store and bought six identical dinner services and six sets of cutlery because I had decided on the spur that I was going to set up my own pop-up restaurant. Now I was in the business of relaxing. Sometimes I did nothing at all.

8. Keeping it inside. Letting it go via writing had been the main thing that had helped me get over drink. No more caging it up, now I had a way to release it.

9. Worrying about the future. The future was going to happen no matter what, and sitting worrying about it was going to solve nothing at all. The best thing was to enjoy the present, I had found, and to savour every blessed moment of being sober and strong. When I started stressing about the future, I put up a big red stop sign.

10. Not looking after myself properly. Mentally,

physically, emotionally. It had to stop, this running myself down the street with a big stick every damn day. It was a new project to replace the drinking lifestyle.

Day 46
Apology to me.

Dear Me,

At the moment you are feeling pretty sorry for yourself what with being ill again this week, probably because of stress. You need to drink more water and get plenty of rest. I want to apologise to you for a few things I have done to you over the years and to reassure you that from now on things are going to be different.

I am sorry for …

– Drinking to the point of you blacking out over many years.

– Not respecting you by eating rubbish food, smoking, and not drinking enough water.

– Making foolish decisions about past and present relationships which led to you getting damaged.

– Allowing others to make decisions for you which made you unhappy.

– Dismissing your feelings because other people had different ones.

– Keeping you quiet about things that were important to you so you didn't rock the boat.

– Not trusting your instincts.

– Spending your money on stupid stuff including alcohol and all the peripherals around alcohol, so now you have nothing.

– Not allowing you time to relax and allowing hurry sickness to take over because stopping still would mean having to think.

– Not allowing you time to explore your creative side.

– Not pushing you harder to write.

– Believing that simply because people say things about you they are therefore right about you.

– Believing that your worst feelings about yourself are facts … they are just feelings.

Now that the drinking has stopped and your head is clear, dear me, I hope you will be able to see a way forward from this and start your life properly. Love xxx

Day 47
Drink and love don't go together.

I was on a love thyself mission that week, having spent a lot of time introspecting. I had a desire to just get rid of it all on 'paper' and felt once this was done I could move on.

My love for drink had ruined so many opportunities that I could not begin to say how strongly I felt about never ever letting myself get that vulnerable again by taking a drug that wanted to destroy me. Talk about misjudging a friend! Story of my life.

- Like drink driving any number of times and pure luck not getting done (I was especially ashamed of doing this).
- Like that job interview with the editor of a regional paper when I was seventeen, and turning up with two large gin and tonics on board.
- Like drinking my way through university and scraping a Thora.
- Like marrying a co-dependent alcoholic wife beater and believing he could change for getting on 10 long years.
- Like desperately searching for new relationships which were actually mainly based on drinking although I called it a 'social life' at the time.
- Like having a beautiful Irish Draught silver horse, riding her drunk, falling off, cracking my leg clean in two and having to sell her, and walking around now with a short leg and pins holding my thigh together, and chronic pain in my wonky hip reminding me daily of how alcohol yet again could have killed me.

Don't be sorry for me. I owned up because it was time, not because I was looking for sympathy. I just wanted people to understand, if they were in any doubt, that alcohol did not equal or deserve love.

This was painful in parts to read, but that was only

because I related to it. I needed to explore brutal honesty and get to the heart of the matter without wrapping it up with tissue paper, hearts, and flowers. I felt scared by how vulnerable this clarity was making me feel, but I guessed I had to stare the Drink Demon in the face until she backed away permanently.

For too long I had laughed off my drunken antics as being an extrovert:

- Nude streaking down my street in the small hours was a particularly 'extrovert' event.
- I once wrote "TWAT", four foot high in black marker pen, at 2 a.m. after a session on the newly painted white garage door of a man who had called my friend's daughter names. Stealing skateboards from the local (noisy) skater boys in our street and hiding them in my garage (the boards not the boys) and finding it hilarious in my inebriated state.
- Pulling a knife on a man who allowed his Rottweiler to attack my dog, in a park, all of this threatening behaviour in full view of other walkers.
- Starting a fight in a night club with a man who kept stealing my chair when I was up dancing and laughing in my face.
- Keeping a walking stick by the door, a metal bar in a cigarette packet in my pocket, a heavy chain under the seat of my car, an air rifle under my bed, and a penknife in my bag, because I was convinced I could be attacked at any point (I lived alone during the worst of this paranoia phase).
- Getting road rage with a massive hangover on board and chasing a car until he parked up, then frightening the living daylights out of him, just because he pulled out of a junction too close to me.

Writing this had told me what would happen if I ever went

back to drink. Recounting (some of) the worst elements of my drinking behaviour reminded me exactly how strong it was, which is why I wrote my thoughts every day, because it saved me from the craving. It took as long as it took.

Day 48
Normas and Normans.

I had a conversation with a neighbour who I consider a Norma yesterday. Sometimes we share news over the fence. A couple of weeks ago I told them in passing I was no longer drinking, no biggie, but for some reason they were fascinated:

Neighbour: Hey, Binki, I have to tell you this. I had a dry weekend last weekend! *(Looks expectant)*

Binki: *(Thinking, what do you want, a coconut? Plus, thanks yet again for reminding me how weird I am for not drinking)* Wow, that's excellent. How did it feel?

Neighbour: *(looks triumphant)* I put on one and a half pounds, that's how it felt. I went to Slimming World on Monday and for the first time since I started, I had put on. So much for not drinking!

Binki: *(thinking, is this my fault?)* Did you maybe eat more than usual? Sugary stuff?

Neighbour: Oh no, I stuck to my plan. But what's the point of not drinking when you put weight on, that's what I'm saying.

Binki: *(imagining dangling neighbour out of the window by her ankles)* Well it was probably water retention … the body does funny things when you stop taking a drug …

Neighbour: Well I'm on the vodka this weekend, and I bet you I lose weight!

Binki: *(please let me win the lottery this weekend)* Enjoy!

I was focusing on wanting to get to that point where it felt right and natural NOT to drink, rather than a massive effort. For the majority of Normas and Normans, like my well- meaning neighbour, drinking was their normal.

I was opting for safe, healthy, and happy Norma. Non-drinking Norma. I didn't want to be digging my garden and tell my neighbour I actually managed not to drink for 48 hours, then went out and got smashed the following weekend and expect them to pat me on the back and say well done. I wanted them to look at me and say fucking hell, that woman doesn't drink, that's amazing. I want to be like her.

Day 49
Feeling optimistic.

I had the usual Friday evening wishful thinking: if only I could have a little snifter …

But following the action of the first drink through to the ultimate denouement of headache, nerves, idle sitting around, feeling sorry for myself, and the pure irritation of having done it, were all putting me off. If I gave in tonight I would regret it. Wobble away, but don't fall.

I didn't know much at all about life and I had messed up so many times no amount of showers and baths would rinse it off me (maybe in the future), but I had got far enough to know that if you stopped, you changed your life. If you don't, you don't.

I still regularly consumed what felt like my whole body weight in chocolate and the Sugar Monster was my next target after the Drink Demon. But it was so damn exciting to be creating this whole new future, having space to grow and change … rather than the slow, predictable, scary, depressing descent of alcohol addiction.

I was stunned that I had arrived at my 49th AF day. I never dreamed I would ever last this long. I wanted to shout from the rooftops, 'If I can do 49 days, anyone can!'

Day 50
The pros and cons of insomnia.

I loved Al Pacino. He was great in *Insomnia* and really all his films did it for me. One of the things I did when lying awake at night in fact was trying to name all the Al Pacino films I had seen and the order I liked them in. Then I tried to identify flags of the world. Or maybe plan how I was going to lose a bit more weight. Then I started thinking about the blasted speeding ticket that I needed to pay (35 mph in a 30 zone. Oops.). And the council tax. And the water bill. Washing the terriers' bedding. If anyone had won the quarter million on *Deal or No Deal* recently. The point of anti-depressants when they seemed to keep me awake.

One thing I didn't think about was what breed of alcohol I was going to consume that coming day. That was a pro of insomnia, waking up and knowing that I wouldn't be drinking that day, even if I had woken up three hours earlier than I needed to. The problem was, I felt so excited and flipping great about not being a drinker any more that my body and mind could not settle into it. I just wanted everyone who was struggling to join the party. It would be the best party they ever went to, even if they did end up a bit short on the sleep side of things. A friend suggested coming round with her remedy: a litre of lavender oil and a mallet!

I was pretty sure it was the fluoxetine causing this madness, ironically. I had doubled my dose in the last couple of weeks and it had been too much of a coincidence that I was now some sort of nocturnal creeping animal. I would go back to the docs … again … the joys of being a middle-aged woman. I had always been an erratic sleeper, but to be honest, even with just a few hours, I still felt better than a night of tossing and turning and panicking and thinking I was going to die of whatever was giving me grief at that moment due to consuming a bottle of wine. I just had to get up in these early weeks and sit with a mutt or two cuddled in on the sofa, because I got so wound up by all the thoughts racing around in my head. Lying awake made them worse, so it was coffee, sunrise, and my hairy terriers, and writing.

Day 51
Real life interfering with my new life.

I loved being in my bubble these past 7-8 weeks. I hoped that soon I could start to just 'be' a non-drinker rather than concentrate entirely on it all hours of the day (and night). It was proving trickier than I thought, though, and I admitted to feeling pretty dependent on writing stuff down.

I told someone I was not drinking any more yesterday and haven't done for getting on for two months. She was a bit taken aback. An event is coming up where everyone will be drinking except me – hope I am wrong. I am dreading it. I found myself justifying my non drinking to this person, a bit like I sometimes ended up justifying my reasons for not having kids (often women in particular think this very personal question is OK to ask even on casual acquaintance and that they are entitled to an honest answer).

So real life was invading my hermit's space.

Then for Saturday, OH has bought tickets for a gig by a band we both love. Normally I would be there dancing away pissed and 'happy' (until the 3 a.m. shakes), but this time I would be sober, and probably driving. What a babe rocker I was. At least I wouldn't get the urge to go out and smoke and flirt with very young men who invite me back to their hotel while hubby was inside the venue wondering where the hell I was …

OH sensed I was getting agoraphobic about the approaching weekend. I hoped I didn't have a meltdown again but I often found real-life situations out of the safe zone. I was so aware that my grip on this AF was fragile and it wouldn't have taken much for me to tip, like tonight when I was tired and stressed. Yet other days I was steady as a rock. This was how recovery went.

Day 52
Normalasaurus rex.

A dear friend who had a bit of a binge recently emailed me saying she was back up on her hind legs again and not drinking. She said she was glad to be normal again. For anyone who was already normal and never gave it a second thought, that was probably a weird thing to say. Fancy not feeling normal. Cheers for the empathy. But as someone who had been in the land of the non-normal for years, decades even, it was a syndrome I could identify with instantly. I too wanted to be seen as 'normal'.

Some people might argue that there was no such thing as normal and abnormal. We all had our own reality and what we thought of as perfectly acceptable was going to feel pretty unusual to someone else. I could not speak for all ex-drinkers, but I did know that as soon as an ex-drinker said they were glad to be normal, I could relate their comment to a whole set of experiences which only me and other addicts could understand. There was barely any explaining to do; it was almost a secret code. The prize of normal.

Normal meant not drinking. Normal meant feeling like a whole person rather than a shell. It meant not being ashamed anymore about my breath, skin, injuries, police involvement, debt, abuse by others, or failed relationships.

It meant not walking into an ordinary supermarket peopled by normals and instantly casing the joint to see what alcohol was on offer, or where to find the cheapest deal in the wine/spirits section, or getting twitchy in case my husband forgot I needed to take the trolley down the drinks aisle before we left, or worrying I hadn't enough money in my purse to get my fix, or planning how I would secretly buy more alcohol later because there wasn't enough in the basket.

Normal meant being able to face people and say ‘I don’t drink’, and feeling so proud I could burst.

Day 53
The answer was always there …

If you looked hard enough. Life became full of ponderables once you stopped drinking, I found, and all sorts of choices popped up which weren't there before, some good, some not so good. For instance, I was worried sick about my OH being out of work and the slow slide we faced to financial ruin. He applied for jobs every day and barely got an acknowledgement, and our relationship was under such strain as a result even though we were deeply in love, and he qualified for absolutely no support from anywhere because I earned my modest wage … enough to send anyone to the bottle … but I hadn't.

I was facing up to this ponderable, as usual in the middle of the night, thinking actually some kind of oriental water torture would be preferable to this insomnia lark, then it suddenly came to me I have been missing a trick. I thought of the solution and felt a whole weight lifting off, and the optimism came back, and once again I felt strong enough to not drink, or rather to carry on not drinking. So when I saw him tonight to talk, we would make some plans to get him registered with lots of recruitment agencies and see where this idea went.

If there really were karma in this world then I hoped we were due a break. Whenever I felt under pressure about money I always tried to think about all the things I had to be thankful for and it did put it in perspective. I even reminded myself that being able to turn on a tap was a luxury. It was true; I was rich in many ways. I had done the having money but unhappy personal life bit and would rather have no money but be in love, (although ideally I'd be rich and be in love, but hey ho). There were always choices, the bottle being a bad one. It was tough times out there, but I had sobriety and the person I loved and who loved me. I was rich, really.

Day 54
A list of cheerfulness.

There is a game is where you have a tray of things, let the children look at it, memorise it, then take it away and return it with some things missing that they need to identify, and the winner is the person getting it right. Maybe it's a teacher thing. That game reminded me of the comment a friend said about remembering all the things that we have to be grateful for and positive about – even when some 'items' are taken away there was still a lot on our trays to be thankful for. They rather sardonically added 'I bet if a bottle was removed from my tray it would be the first thing I noticed … '

Reasons to be cheerful:

1. The people who love us and loved us when we were drunk and didn't leave us but stuck it out and were patient and kind.
2. The air that we are free to breathe and the space we are free to move about in.
3. The choices we can make every day for ourselves without interference or influence by other addicts.
4. The clear head we wake up with in the morning.
5. The feeling of excitement when we realise life is going to be a lot simpler today with no alcohol to balance.
6. The extra time we have now that we don't drink and the time to explore our new selves (or the old self that was poorly).
7. The fresh desire to get creative in whatever sphere we favour.
8. The plans we can enjoy making and the dreams we can look forward to fulfilling because we don't drink any more.
9. The things we are capable of physically because we are fit and healthy (or at least fitter and healthier).

10. The way we look and feel and the appreciation of this by others.

It was amazing to think people could take just one thing away (alcohol) from life's 'tray' and gain so much in return. There really was so much to be grateful for.

Day 55
A middle-aged weeble beating the Friday wobble.

Hit week 8 tomorrow, yay! The time was flying by and so much had happened in a 'mental' sense. A lot of ex-drinkers had Friday wobbles, and I was writing like mad in my journal to gain strength to combat the urges and the panic, which I still got even then, although it was getting easier as the pattern of not drinking repeated itself more and more often. Weebles wobble but they don't fall down (that won't make sense to anyone in their twenties probably).

This Friday was going to be a bit more of a potential wobble for me as I had to go to a work do following a training day; people at work have been talking about it all week. But every time I heard this do mentioned I felt sick with nerves because I hated standing out to start with, was still the newbie of the company, and would be clearly not drinking while everyone else would.

OH said not to worry, they will understand you are driving and as they are nice people they won't judge, but I was still going to feel like an outsider.

Took a sleeping tablet for the first time in my life last night as this insomnia thing was just out of control, and I did sleep like a baby, but it seemed with these new tablets, my anti-ds, and painkillers for this leg of mine that gives me chronic gip, I was just a human pill bottle. Take care of you, as Davina said (a wonderful sober lady).

Day 56
Friday 13th wasn't unlucky.

I counted myself very lucky for lots of reasons this evening, returning from a 14-hour day. Talk about a test of stamina.

I was lucky because:

- I didn't drink and made this fact public and was not struck down.
- I worked with nice people who may not fully understand but did accept that I had made a choice.
- I wouldn't wake up with a hangover from hell tomorrow like my (some of) my workmates who were just getting warmed up when I left them at 10.30 p.m.
- I could go out and not get blasted and make a tit of myself and it felt OK.
- I made better conversation and charmed people rather than annoyed them when I didn't drink.
- I spent less than a fiver on drinks (work funded our meal, bless them).
- I was proud to be strong and independent enough not to fall in with the crowd without considering my options, and was looking after myself properly for the first time in decades.
- People liked and responded positively to me as sober me.
- I could be daft and have ridiculous conversations without being pissed and it was still fun to muck about.
- I still had my sobriety intact and cherished it more than ever.

I realised that if I had drank tonight, I would have been writing full of remorse, self-hatred, and guilt. I knew my OH would say I wouldn't have let him down but it meant a lot to me that I have stayed sober and hopefully showed people who may be wobbling that it was possible, it could be done, just ride it out.

In many ways tonight was the biggest deal of my non-drinking life so far; I had been ill with nerves and apprehension, but I did it, and I had fear still at various points, but I could honestly say I never once looked at the glasses of fizz surrounding me and thought, please give me some of that. It looked fetid. The sound of drunken people on the streets was pathetic. The many police cars scooting about and the general air of violence made me angry. I was not part of that world any more; I left it behind in July, and having been there, done it, and got the T-shirt I was going to treasure my new found Better Life.

When I looked back I wondered what I was afraid of in stopping. Some people did feel they could quiz you – they usually had a problem themselves. In the past I was pretty dismissive of non-drinkers myself and assumed they were very dull. If I'd ever taken off the blinkers and gotten to know any then I'd have discovered some splendid people.

I was just so glad I managed a night with drinkers and didn't join in, if that made sense. I was drinking Red Bull, sparkling water, and fresh orange last night and enjoyed each one. I did relax myself and had some very refreshingly silly conversations too, but the last time I went on a work do with a different company I got smashed, went round every bloke in the room asking for a Christmas kiss, and was so drunk I actually could not speak when my poor OH picked me up.

Day 57
Learning to be alone.

Tonight I tried and failed to go to a simple bloody gig in town, having had a panic attack on the way to the venue and confusing and upsetting my husband, who didn't know what was going on and didn't know how to help. I just couldn't put one foot in front of the other; it was like I was made of cement. My head was thumping and I felt like I might faint. I felt pathetic and scared. He didn't know what to do with me generally, what with all those tablets I was taking, the non-drinking struggle, not speaking to my family, the money crap we had, his guilt at not having a job … a big mess.

It struck me that I had to learn to deal with this stuff mainly on my own because other people just could not be in my head, and I needed to learn how to deal with it in a way that was least scary and upsetting for observers.

I didn't feel alone talking to people online but I didn't half feel lonely in 'real' life, even despite the man who adored me and wanted to help. Being sober was a lonely business in many ways, because the biggest friend I thought I had, the Drink Demon, turned out to be a two-faced liar and not my friend at all.

Early sobriety was a very fragile thing. I had forgotten how humans work as I poisoned myself for so long. The first whiff of anxiety led to wine. Only now did I see the withdrawal caused the anxiety. I have researched and tried to self-practice some CBT for my wonky brain and it has helped.

It was hard to accept I had been and was still poorly, but I was coming out of it now and I was going to achieve so much in the years ahead. I had to get used to listening to my gut, trusting my instincts, and having myself as a friend. Once-familiar situations now felt all wrong and disjointed. Perhaps my new awareness and subsequent revulsion at my past was what was causing the panic attacks. My body was just saying 'No!'

Following advice, I made a nice cuppa, sat down, put my feet up, and just tried to get it all in perspective. I had a bit of a panic attack; it happened to a lot of people. I was amazed that was all that happened, given what I had been through in the last few weeks. I was clearly still coping with the effects of withdrawal, had mental-health problems, and was struggling with money. As time passed these attacks would lessen and the bad days would be replaced by great days.

I hoped for the day I would not give a shit about drinking, or other people drinking. My main hope was that when I gave up regular smoking a while ago, it took me a fair old while to get past the feeling of occasionally wanting a cig; the thing was I had the fabulous benefits of being a non-smoker, and I didn't want to lose that, so didn't want to resume smoking. My giving up drinking experience was a bit similar. These days I was never tempted to smoke, so I reckoned the day would come when I would not care about booze.

Even when I was knocking back vast quantities of wine, cider, and lager, I never really liked pubs and would only truly want to go if I was already at the 'too pissed to be legally served' stage and/or the booze had run out at home. They were often just stinky places filled with drunken assholes (like my old self). Now I was sober I could see that my distaste of pubs was one of the few things I had ever seen clearly through the wine fog. Nothing wrong with avoiding them for the rest of my life, then!

I ragged my husband during this panic attack thing, whatever it was, and called him names, which was so stupid as he was so kind and loving and he was completely bewildered by my freak-out. However I apologised and things were OK again. It was easy to forget that the people we loved had to go through our recovery too.

I was not sure when we would be out again in town; it just felt wrong being out in and around pubs and stuff when I hated the smell and look of drink, even being near drinkers, but friends advised there would come a time when I didn't give a shit. I realised the feeling of being surrounded by drunk people was part of what sparked me off. Please hurry up, don't-give-a-shit feeling!

Day 58
Saluting the power of rambling.

So, life carried on, after a shoddy attempt at a pleasant night out. I went back to my routine from the early days of my recovery, where I spent most of my days tramping about with the mutts, to take my mind off evening drinking.

I would like to recommend walking as therapy, not just because of its ability to tone you up and slim you down, but because mentally I have found it straightened me out quicker than practically any other remedy.

It didn't matter where I rambled, for how long, or with whom/what. The results were always the same. By the time I got back in the house I felt refreshed and ready to carry on. It was such a great distraction from stressful and annoying things going on, and forced me to focus on the simple act of putting one foot in front of the other to the exclusion of all my other worries.

There were no special clothes or equipment to buy and it cost not a jot. A dog (even an ugly one and/or a borrowed one) and/or a good human companion (looks also didn't matter) then so much the better, but company wasn't necessary to still feel the benefits.

So I would continue to ramble away, in my journal and on my paws, especially the next time I felt the pull of the drink. By the time I walked it out, the addiction had crawled back under its rock. Wishing you happy feet also.

We had howling gales with heavy squalls and hail yesterday and today. Never let it be said I was not a conscientious dog owner – poor mutts got dragged out whether they wanted to go or not. There was a lovely area near where I lived that was full of challenging hills and woods. I hadn't been all summer so it was the first time back today. I couldn't wait; it lifted my spirits and knackered me at the same time. I twittered on to myself all the way round (well I pretended I was talking to the dogs), but my excuse was, I was 47 years old; I was old enough to do as I liked.

Day 59
Weird shit I don't do any more.

Looking back on my drinking years, I did some really weird things. For years and years. Repeatedly.

- Drinking, obviously.
- Ordering stuff from catalogues that I didn't want or need and that were completely useless to me.
- Going out on dates with (and on one occasion marrying) people I didn't find attractive.
- Eating food that when sober looked like something I wouldn't give to my dogs.
- Buying 'friendship' and 'love' with gifts and favours and submissive behaviour.
- Gossiping when it was bound to backfire and cause me more harm than the subject.
- Getting into debt by buying duplicates of things I already had and didn't like the first time I bought them either.
- Constantly moving house.
- Constantly changing jobs.
- Using the above as an excuse not to stay still and therefore have to face facts.
- Believing it was a fact when people said I would never stick at anything and acting it out.
- Saying yes when I meant no and no when I meant yes, over important stuff too.
- Making allowances for bullies.
- Buying clothes that didn't fit.
- Buying gym memberships and not going. For years.
- Being friends with people I didn't actually like because the alternative was to be alone and believing the reason I didn't like them was because there was something wrong with me/my attitude, when actually we just weren't suited.

- Jumping into situations, impetuously, for the hell of it, without thinking about the fallout.
- Spending money uselessly and relentlessly.

I knew this all sounded crackers but I didn't want sympathy. I just wanted to list it. I was experiencing puzzlement over my various behaviours and not for a minute assuming I was the only person who had done weird stuff while leading a drinking lifestyle, but I just didn't get why I had been on this mission to self-destruct for so long.

The reason I felt like writing it down was because tonight I went on a catalogue website thinking I would spend a pile of money on credit to make myself feel better, but it felt wrong and strange, not comforting at all as it would have been if I had been sitting with a glass of wine while I did it. So I came off the site, having failed to find the elusive high, and wrote in my journal instead, affording myself a heavy dose of empowerment instead of more debt.

I was OK to admit that somehow, somewhere along the way, I let alcohol have more power over me than it should have done. I wasn't a really bad person with terrible secrets. Instead I was actually an all right person who developed a nasty habit.

I reckoned the biggest, the most wonderful thing about not drinking was the return of self-esteem and confidence, and the massive highs and lows of emotion that were beginning to meet somewhere nearer the middle. My emotions seemed to be more on an even keel those days, rather than the roller coaster I was on when I was drinking every day. The other thing that helped my progress beyond any measure was the way my self-esteem improved when I could successfully say 'no'.

My stomach churned just reading back that list. They say your life passed before your eyes when you had a near-death experience – I thought the drunken me must be in the process of dying as I was currently living with all my past misdemeanors flying in front of my face on a daily basis. Not a comfortable experience, but I let the stomach churn, closed my eyes, breathed deeply, allowed the panic to die, and it all confirmed even more strongly than ever why I needed to stay sober.

I would have liked to say the thoughts went away sooner or later. But at the oddest of times something I didn't know I even knew would flash up and gave me a cringe moment. It seemed the longer I went on, the further the memories went back; the good old subconscious having a clear out. The reassuring thing was that if I practised often enough, I could acknowledge the memories, have a cringe, but know it was done and I couldn't go back and change anything, so move on. I was training myself to succeed.

I knew now it was really dumb to:

- Ask someone who has already told you they aren't drinking at the moment if they want a drink.
- Suggest to someone who doesn't want to drink that they could just have one.
- Get annoyed because someone isn't joining in with drinking – what does it matter to you anyway?
- Look down on non-drinkers as if they are somehow off the team because they don't do this drug any more.
- Suggest that next time they could leave the car at home so they can 'go on the drink', as if taking the car was an unfortunate situation they could have got out of with a bit more organization.
- Feel sorry for people who don't drink because they cannot possibly enjoy themselves at any point.
- Moan about being fat and then sink wine at 150

calories a glass x 2 bottles (about 1400 cals).

- Spend a fortune on healthy foods/boot camps/gym memberships/spa days/diet websites and still drink like a fish.

It was time to cringe again as I read this back, as I knew I was guilty of so many of them. I remembered a gang of us spiking someone's drinks on his 21st; the poor guy was so ill he was lucky he didn't end up in hospital. I remember also buying a friend treble whisky and cokes as a joke instead of the singles she requested, only for her to be chucking up in and consequently thrown out of a taxi on the way home because she was being ill all over his back seat. So she had to sit on a roundabout island and do it in full view of the traffic instead, and it was all my fault.

Oh yes – my old favourite was the supplements to counteract the drinking. I would quaff a bottle of wine every night and it would be OK because I would take a shed load of milk thistle and vitamins in the morning and slap some really expensive cream on with tons of foundation to hide the redness on my nose and cheeks and the big black bags under my eyes …

Dumb things I used to say, part two:

- I need to drink. If I don't drink, I won't be able to cope.
- Drinking is the only thing that cheers me up.
- Drinking relieves my stress and makes me feel better.
- Drinking is purely a social activity, enabling me to communicate better with my peers.
- Drinking makes me feel attractive and lovable.
- Drinking cements friendships and work partnerships.
- Drinking makes me feel young again.

- Drinking is all I have to look forward to.
- Drink is my friend.
- Drinking makes me a better person.
- Drinking gives me the confidence to be a nutter.
- Drinking means I achieve far more in my life than I ever anticipated.
- Drinking means I don't have to communicate with anyone normally.
- Drinking means I don't have to have feelings.
- Drinking is my life.

Day 60
Clever things non-drinkers say.

So the week was travelling inexorably towards Friday again, that tricky time which no matter how many weeks in to AF I got, I still got a massive twinge at around 6 p.m. when traditionally I would have cracked open the red and got steadily sloshed, only to wake at 3 a.m. feeling like I had been in an accident. Then I'd spend Saturday a bundle of hangover nerves, waiting for Saturday wine o'clock to make it disappear.

So I tried to say clever things to myself to stop the build-up to Friday night being such a big deal. These are things I have read and heard wiser non-drinkers than me say that soothed and relaxed and strengthened my resolve:

- I am making a positive choice not to drink.
- I am looking forward to having a great day with a clear head tomorrow.
- I impress my loved ones and I love the look in their eyes when they see me not drinking.
- I am actually rewarding myself with my fave treats rather than buying stuff just to make myself feel better.
- My body is functioning better and people tell me I look better these days.
- I believe I can do things that weren't possible before.
- The world has become a more exciting place.
- I don't need alcohol to have a good time.
- I don't need the people who require me to be vulnerable to be successful in life, or to have their approval in order to exist. I don't fit in the box/compartment they have chosen for me any more.
- I don't need to exhaust myself trying to be someone I am not. I can 'not like' some stuff and 'like' other stuff and it is OK.

- It is OK to be still and contemplative and not do much at all.
- It is OK to just be.

Day 61
Help often comes from unexpected quarters.

I was so grateful for all the help I had had. Being able to help others also helped me get to where I was; part of a nice big loving friendship circle. It struck me too how help comes from the most unlikely of sources – who would have thought a website of anons would offer so many like-minded people so much hope and a future?

My husband, who was still out of work, received a match ticket and a tenner through the post for a Balti pie and a Bovril at the match next week, from an online friend on a forum he chats on about footie. Not something he asked for, but a generous gift from a well-wisher out of the blue who just wanted him to have a break from this relentless hell called unemployment.

It reminded me also of 11 years ago, when I had to spend 6 months in the house recovering from my broken leg, the secretary of the school I worked for at the time filled my fridge and did my other shopping for me for several weeks, without prompting, and was so kind and non-judgmental, while my drinking 'buddies' were all of a sudden strangely absent.

So it was always surprising who was there for you when you most needed it, and help would always come from unexpected quarters. I still had my faith in the basic good in human nature, despite so much evidence to the contrary. Kindness was a wonderful thing. Now that I was less snappy and impatient and generally angry with the world and myself, I was hoping to show more of my own good nature to others in return for kindnesses received.

There was a magnificent moon shining tonight which nearly matched the glow in my heart for managing to still stay off the drink, helped along by the unexpected kindness of others both now and as memories, which warmed the cockles, as they say.

Day 62
Outing with the folks.

We stopped at my folks' for some moussaka and cake (not at the same time) and my mother kindly offered me a glass of wine with my lunch, a gesture which amused me, but only a few weeks ago would have sent me up the wall.

Instead of annoyance my overwhelming feeling was one of pride, hopefully not in an arrogant way; it was rather like being in a huge balloon, bowling down a hill, bouncing off the stones lightly and without discomfort, being caught up by the wind, looking at amazing views of valleys and mountains, and experiencing an incredible sense of freedom. I don't drink, thank you.

Our meal with my parents followed a day in the Lake District, where we drove over the Honister Pass in 70 mph winds, the rain pelting down and our tiny red car almost lifting off the road. We had to drive up the wrong side of the little road to avoid being driven over the sheer edge into the rocky ravine below, where we would be hidden from any rescuers' view by trees and shrubs. It was a daft and dangerous thing to do, but the pure exhilaration of conquering that summit despite the odds, playing AC/DC's 'Hells Bells' as we descended, reminded me of the liberation of finding I am no longer dependent on alcohol.

I found myself making comparisons with risks in life and the risks involved in giving up my 'friend' alcohol. In the past I often thought I was safe when I was actually doing something very dangerous. I was lulled into a false sense of security by the knowledge that I was doing something familiar, but actually I was harming myself. Drinking alcohol with abandon over thirty odd years, for me put any risk offered by the Honister Pass into perspective.

Day 63
Nine weeks.

Nine weeks with me would be enough to drive anyone nuts, ha-ha.

I needed to tell others how worth it was to see out the bad times and get to the point where it felt natural and normal to CHOOSE not to drink.

So nine weeks. I wondered what would happen at nine and a half weeks. The Friday attack from the Drink Demon would still happen to me at around 3 p.m. – 6 p.m. the same as it did every week, and I would have my usual mini strop in my head where I had to flop out on the bed and grumble because I wanted to get pissed, then I would remind myself of all my journal entries and life would go on.

Not in a million years did I ever dream I would get this far. The first few weeks I felt terrified and sick with worry. Looking back I have now worked out why I was so scared. The Drink Demon had damaged me so much I knew that this was the last chance saloon; I couldn't afford for this attempt to fail … I knew I would be finished.

I felt I had every smug right to feel victorious, clever, talented, and strong. There were days that I was literally giddy with the knowledge that I was not imprisoned by alcohol. It was such a pleasure to be in this state of mind.

The key for me was not telling yourself you could not drink, but instead telling yourself you could if you wanted, but you chose not to. I had to approach it this way. I was choosing something. I was not denying myself anything. I could have a drink anytime I want. But I didn't want to … so there!

Day 64
Wishing alcohol would just fuck off.

I got through that Friday's wobble, though I was not helped by listening to people obsessing over details of what they planned to drink that weekend.

It really struck home listening to these people, who really didn't deserve my bitter thoughts – who am I to judge them anyway? – that I had literally not physically touched a bottle or a can of alcohol with my hands since packing in and actually the thought of doing so made me twitchy. So I was not out of the woods, even after all those weeks.

I thought because I worked in the challenging situations I did, I witnessed the effects of a lot of drug and alcohol abuse by vulnerable people, and it sickened me but at the same time I am ashamed to admit I felt relieved that it wasn't me and I had been lucky enough not to sink any further.

I was very open with the learners at work about not drinking and had discussions at length with many of them. I was also open about my decision to stop drinking with my work colleagues and others I came into contact with – I was proud of being a non-drinker. The time for being secretive was when I was drinking heavily and behaving in ways I found cringeworthy in retrospect, although I realised that at the time, I was far more mentally damaged than I knew.

I had a learner the other day who said he used to be an alcoholic but now he only drinks eight cans a night, and he wasn't joking. I had another one yesterday who asked if I was going out on the drink this weekend and I explained I don't drink, he said why not? I told him that I had realised I had a problem with it, and he accepted it but 'the look' was still in his eyes. I regularly had learners come in the morning smelling of stale drink, and people even came for interviews for our courses with drink on them. I really was looking forward not to giving a shit about what other people drank and how it may or may not affect me, but the line of work I was in and the attitudes up here in the North East of the UK meant that I was constantly exposed to it and really did wish I could get through a day without someone intruding my personal space with it.

I had been upset to read my upsetness in the early days of my diary; it seemed as if it was a different person and that person is someone I should be writing a comforting comment to. At the time, in the early weeks, wiser people than me told me that one day:

- The issues that made me cry would not do so any more.
- I wouldn't care what people thought of me not drinking.
- The gaping time slots that had opened up would be filled with something more interesting than interacting with a Drink Demon.
- I would feel like being more creative than I ever had in my life.
- I would look forward rather than back all the time.
- Memories would not hurt me.
- Feelings are not facts.
- I would forgive myself and others.
- I would go out and have fun without the Drink Demon.

The wise friends were right. Which is why it was so important to remember that real history was being made for every person who got sober; the start of something very powerful and real. We could all be a part of the growth of sober life and make it happen, sooner rather than later.

Day 65
Mrs Serenity.

I decided to be calm and serene today, perusing my world and ignoring the chaos. That was the beauty of AF. You chose to be who you wanted, without alcohol dictating the measure of your day.

I did an 8-mile stroll with the terriers and OH yesterday afternoon, beautiful sunshine, no wind, leaves changing colour, and felt at peace. We sat on a bench outside Sainsbury's half way round, at a point where weeks ago I might have popped in and bought a bottle or some cans to take home, ignoring the way the carrier bag cut into my hand as I walked home with it. As we sat on the bench we estimated that maybe 90% of the shoppers coming in and out had some form of drink in their arms. Openly and without giving a stuff, crates and crates of it. It was normal to drink to excess. I couldn't change that.

But I could join a revolution, at least amongst people of the same mind. The bigger world was a different matter. But in my own life, my own communications, with my own loved ones and on my own, I could change my own world.

My OH had hardly touched a drop since I went AF. He described 'beer fear' and talked about the immense amount of binge drinking he had done over the years to stave off boredom, be one of the lads, to try and forget depression and a horrible family life; for all kinds of reasons. I was so proud of him and going AF had made us stronger. I was sure he would have a pint or two at some point, but just then he didn't care two hoots about it, would rather have a chilled coke in his special Guinness pint glass. So I was going to follow the example set by his coke and chill today. I might be going crackers again tomorrow, but at least I would be sober doing it.

Being AF made me see the world in a whole new light.

Simple pleasures meant a lot more to me now than before and although I had still done some of the 'old style' socialising, I had to come home early as all my friends, who I did really love, started to talk crap and laugh at nonsense.

I found people were talking to me about how they'd like to really cut down. So many people were not really enjoying it any more. I tried to tell them, there were so many other things that could make them happy – all precious and all free.

Day 66
Returning to simple pleasures.

Life with alcohol in it seemed very complicated; all that organising and planning and making sure of supply. It was so refreshing to wake up and get a little frisson because life was going to be pretty straightforward in the day, and pleasant at night. The annoying stuff/people still happened, but they could be dealt with in a way that they never could be before. I used to stew and ruminate for hours about the most idiotic situations when actually it was just a case of shrugging and moving on.

As part of life getting simpler I was happy to revisit simple pleasures which I denied myself when drinking was more important.

1. Cycling. Getting on a bike and going out in the sun for a pedal.

2. Smiling at people who smiled back, or returning smiles from people instead of focusing on my busting head.

3. Walking a long way. Exercising the mutts was too often a hasty chore to get out the way, and yet I would spend hours sitting with a drink by my side watching crap on the goggle box. Now I walked twice as far in a day and longer at weekends. The benefits of walking made a long list on their own.

4. Writing. Most of it was nonsense that only I could decipher but it gave me such a great break from reality.

5. Painting. I was not a very good artist and never would be, but I loved creating little watercolours and had never had the patience to sit still for long enough to do it when alcohol was around.

6. Watching a good film. Like painting, I couldn't sit still and concentrate on a film all the way through, or else I would fall asleep as a result of the drink and miss the end.

7. Reading. Oh how I adored reading. I have always

loved a good story and for years now neglected this simple pleasure. Being in bed all snuggled – and conscious – with a book to read was sooo good.

8. Talking. My OH was telling me today how it felt to be on the receiving end of my drunken blabbing; I hated hearing it but needed to. I didn't think I had as many interesting conversations in all the years I drank as I have in recent weeks.

9. Thinking. It was great to be able to think and come to a conclusion, instead of thinking about stuff, forgetting it, coming back to it, forgetting it again, and deciding it wasn't worth thinking about in the first place.

10. Feeling. I decided I was probably mad as a hatter and had been for a while, but actually I didn't feel bad about that any more. It was just how I was. I didn't need to squash it, or be ashamed of it, or try and fit in with others people's views of how I should be/change. This thing of 'why don't you …' which seemed to echo round me throughout my life was no longer relevant to me. It seemed there was a common denominator of feeling a bit mad in people who had beaten an addiction. Maybe it was the feeling of release from their alter egos, the permission to be who they really were and the pure crazy joy of having been able to do it.

There was also the crazy joy that came with the understanding that there was a chance to make up for lost time; to make full use of what I had and have some bliddy fun for a change. For instance, I realised how little smiling I did sometimes and was trying to change that, even if people thought I was simple. Most people did respond positively! I had also been reading about two books a week since going AF, doing yoga, playing my favourite music again and taking my dogs on endless walks. It was shocking how alcohol just ate into time.

Day 67
How to take care of yourself during a bad day.[1]

1. Recognise that needing to drink is a feeling. There are always underlying emotions that we attach to drinking. When the 'I need a drink' thoughts start up, try to identify what you're feeling underneath the craving. Are you feeling lonely? Anxious? Inadequate? Invisible? Scared? Ashamed? Bored? Whatever the feelings are, recognise that they are separate from you.

2. Treat yourself as you would a friend. Because it's difficult to be kind to ourselves in the moment when the self-hating thoughts take over, try responding to your thoughts as if you were supporting a friend. What would you say to someone you loved who was battling your same struggle with drinking? You wouldn't tell them to drink more in order to compensate for what they drank the previous night. You wouldn't tell them to punish themselves for their drinking through self-harm, or abusive habits. You wouldn't tell them they were worthless or unlovable because of their drinking. So why do you tell yourself these things? Break the cycle and start treating yourself like a friend – you deserve that kindness and love from everyone, especially yourself.

3. Recognise that you are so much more than your drinking. What you drink does not define you. It doesn't discount your worth as a human being. As a living, breathing, feeling human being you have inherent value. You are special and important and loved. Your addiction is such a small part of who you are, and it certainly doesn't

---

[1] I do not claim this information entirely as my own, I have edited it from a pin on my Pinterest page courtesy of the internal-acceptance-movement. Hope it helps and thank you to them for posting it online.

warrant enough power to discount the person you are inside. You aren't your addiction – you are your goals and dreams and passions and values. You are your strengths and talents and insight. You are a soul and a spirit and a force of nature. Your drinking habit does not define you.

4. Shift your focus from the external to the internal. Make a list of all the people you look up to and are inspired by – not because of their ability to take a drink, but because of who they are and what they do. Write out all the qualities they have that make you appreciate and value them. Use the list as a reminder that it's the internal things – our dreams and passions and goals and morals and insight and character – that truly define who we are and draw people to us; not our drinking. You are no exception to this. Try making your own list of things you like about yourself that have nothing to do with alcohol. If you have a difficult time creating one, ask some friends and family to help you.

5. Think about what you want to be remembered for after you die. I don't want people to remember me for what I was like when I was drunk. I want to be remembered for the person I am. I want to be remembered as someone who brought about positive change in the world. I want to be remembered as loving friend, partner, and family member. I want to be remembered for my passions and my creativity and my strength. I want to be remembered as someone who made a difference. What do you want your legacy to be? Chances are, it doesn't have anything to do with alcohol.

6. Instead of focusing on your craving for drink, start focusing on what your body allows you to do. The human body is an incredible force. When we get caught up in the number on the scale and size of clothes however, we forget just how lucky we are to have a fully functioning vehicle to engage in life with. So stop abusing and hating your body for the way it looks and start acknowledging and

appreciating your body for all that it allows you to do. Make a list of each activity and feat your body helps you to partake in and accomplish. Your body is strong, powerful, and beautiful, regardless of its size. Choose to treat it with love, compassion, and gratitude instead of pouring alcohol into it.

7. Challenge your negative thoughts. You may not be able to change the way you feel about your drinking today, tomorrow, or a month from now, but you can begin the process by challenging the thoughts in the moment. Write out a dialogue between your negative voice and a healthy AF voice. If you have a hard time coming up with positive counters to the negative thoughts, pretend that you are speaking positively about a friend or loved one. Even if you don't believe the things you say to counter the voice, it's still important to speak out against it, because each time you argue with the thoughts, you are taking away some of their power and reclaiming your own. The more you challenge the thoughts, the less you will believe them.

8. Allow yourself to feel your feelings. There is a lot of built up energy and emotion underlying the way we feel about our bodies. Holding in how we feel or engaging in behaviours to numb out may make us feel better in the moment, but in the long run, it doesn't remedy the pain we feel. It doesn't make us feel better and it keeps us stuck. Releasing the energy and painful emotions underlying our body shame requires us to feel our feelings. Whether that means throwing a tantrum on the floor, venting to a friend on the phone, punching a pillow, screaming in your car, or crying in bed, you need to allow yourself to feel your feelings. Let go of the judgment you have about what you feel and recognise that you are feeling these things for a reason. Give yourself permission to release your emotions and let everything out.

9. Do self-care. When you're struggling with alcohol, distract yourself with healthy coping mechanisms. Take a

bubble bath, ask for a back scratch, cuddle a pet, make plans with a supportive friend, watch your favourite film – whatever it is, make sure it's something self-soothing and helps you get out of your head.

10. Be kind to yourself. You may not be able to control the way you feel about alcohol, but you can control what you do in response to how you feel. Instead of beating yourself up, you can choose to treat yourself with compassion. Instead of engaging in unhealthy and abusive behaviours, you can choose to do self-care. Instead of treating your body as an enemy, you can choose to treat it as a friend. Instead of isolating yourself, you can choose to reach out for support and surround yourself with positive people who make you feel loved and accepted. Instead of agreeing with the negative thoughts, you can choose to challenge them. You have more power than you think – don't let the way you feel about drink keep you from living. Coping with bad days may not be easy, but it is possible. Don't give up. You aren't alone. Things can and will get better.

This information really saved me tonight. It was just what I needed to read. Mostly, the first one; recognise that the need to drink was a feeling. From there I became present and allowed my rational mind to join the conversation with my irrational (alcoholic/ego-based mind) and ask myself, 'What am I feeling that's making me *feel* like I need to drink.' From there I proceeded to make a fattening, decadent fruit cake and gobble it up as soon as it had cooled a little, while pondering my desire to drink. I know that I just replaced the alcohol with the cake but there were worse things I could do. Anyway, I made it through what I thought might have been a huge slip after these last weeks being AF. It's really interesting to ponder the 'why' and the fact that alcohol would not make it better, so why did I sometimes think it would, even for a moment.

I really identified with the idea of being defined by drink. I had got to the stage where I was allowing drink to define me but now I felt really free.

When I argued with my first husband about the fact that he still knocked me about and was lying about various affairs, he would put me down, sometimes literally, and look at me with such utter contempt that I felt I had no choice but to self-medicate. He reduced me to the point at where I felt I was nothing and meant nothing and of course the more useless I felt the more I would turn to wine for comfort and to block out these feelings. Any plonk would do in those desperate circumstances, although when alone I often also drank expensive ones that were being saved for a social event, just for the revenge factor. Then the whole rowing and abuse cycle would start again and I became ever more hobbled and incapable of saving myself.

Of course I realised now I was making the whole sick situation 10 times worse for myself by getting pissed all the time, but I really didn't know what else to do in those days. I knew he had a point about my drinking but he refused to help me because he liked it too much too. He worked long shifts and I suspect was telling he was working even when he didn't have a shift, having one day found a worn dress shirt and tie stuffed under the passenger seat of his car (I was quite the detective by this time), that he certainly hadn't worn out with me. And let's not even go there with the mobile phone and the credit card bills (jewellery, restaurant bills, flowers …), towards the end he did not even try to hide his subterfuge, what a clichéd mess. Or the drunken Christmas day where he phoned my parents and told them to come and collect me as he had had enough of my boozing, when actually it was him that was more steaming than me. They came up on their Christmas Day, an hour's drive, and were bewildered by what they found, and very sad. I was lying in bed, surrounded by tear-soaked tissues, a bottle of brandy on the duvet, face red, mascara blackening my eyes and cheeks, unwashed and stinking. I refused my parents' offers of help. Later, when it was all over, they told me they came close to disowning me that day, they just couldn't take any more.

I also drank the night after I had consulted a solicitor about a possible divorce, when I finally realised things were irretrievable. It wasn't so much the fact that I had decided I wanted a divorce, but the fact that the blond little Sloane who I paid to see, advised me she could not represent me because she had only just realised, after listening to the most intimate details of my marriage, that she already 'knew' my husband. Turns out he had even been there, the dirty fanny rat!

I saw now that actually I was a valid person and deserved to be treated so. I took responsibility for my past actions and excessive drinking and I wished to God I could turn back the clock. At least now though, I had a chance to make a change for the better.

Day 68
We should never feel ashamed.

Someone spoke to me last night in a way that took me back to my childhood at the speed of light, and brought up all kinds of feelings that I had been working very hard to excommunicate from my fragile new life. When one stuck one's head above the parapet and had the courage to reach out to others, there would always be people who sought to jump on your head and stamp you back down into your hole. But I wanted to encourage people to be brave and strong and remember why they were beating addiction in the first place, so I continued to voice my thoughts online, in the same direct manner.

Addiction was very, very clever and would use literally any means to get people to wobble and to consider seeking relief without considering the final outcomes, which were always the same. It will try to undermine the hard work, kill the new self-esteem, and send messages via negative people that drinking wasn't so bad really, and try all means possible to divert its target from the one true course, which was to stop drinking altogether. I had to tell myself 'Don't listen to the negative voices and keep strong.'

I was trying really hard to remember that the real enemy was always alcohol, not the people who carried its messages of addiction. A kind friend who sensed my vulnerability at that point said: 'It is about learning to live with and tolerate other people's behaviour, however irritating or downright unpleasant it may seem to me. It's not worth jeopardising my sobriety over. My recovery is way too important. I can try and understand them, don't have to agree, and try to not get upset by things, but at the end of the day I have to walk away and live my own life, leave them to theirs. You've felt this, and you've done some good dealing and healing.'

Day 69

Keeping a treasure chest.

Someone wiser than me told me once it is a good idea to collect together all the nice things that have happened and the nice things people have said, and put them all in a treasure chest. Then when the walls start closing in and you feel like you are suffocating with the pressure of those walls pushing you into a smaller and smaller space, you can open the lid of the treasure chest and take out those things and those words, and they will make you feel better again.

I had my treasure chest open off and on all day, revisiting the wonderful comments people had made to me, the things people have said to me in life generally. Super stuff like standing on the top of a mountain and feeling the wind in my face, and spits of rain on my skin, and knowing that I am alive and strong. Riding my horse and smelling her scent, and feeling her mane against my cheek when we cuddled. The smiles on my terriers' little furry faces when they saw me coming in the back door and the fact that OH says they sit waiting for me by the door for an hour beforehand, every day. Getting married in the sunshine and seeing love in my partner's eyes. My boss, complimenting my work. None of it had the least thing to do with getting pissed. All those particular memories were crap.

I could recommend having a treasure chest for the times when you were low, or you may have your own version? All you have to do is open up the lid and take the things and the words out one by one, and savour them again, and be glad to be alive and to have had those special experiences. None of it should be anything to do with alcohol. Then you put them back for the next time.

Day 70
Smugger smugly smugathon smug out.

10 weeks 10 weeks 10 weeks 10 weeks. OMG.

Fridays were always dodgy. Although the rest of the week I could pootle on OK and actively despise alcohol, every Friday with the start of the weekend, the old memory of getting out of my head still returned. The feeling of getting to the end of the weekend without a drink was still amazing, and a relief. As long as I got this rollercoaster happening, I still needed to count the days/weeks and be grateful. Once I stopped counting I would know the war was over, but was not sure how long that would take. That after 100 days being AF would just be normal and not something that consumed my every thought and action, as it did at this time. That idea of just having a state of 'being' was on my mind much more these days and I was pleased, as it signified a new stage in my recovery.

I wished the anger would just fuck off, as well. I was angry with the anger! But I was working on it. I was still in the 'why me' stage, but I guessed I would move on eventually. Part of me actually enjoyed ranting though. I mean, if I didn't have something to fight against, what the hell was I supposed to do with my life? Just get on with it?

A friend with a much better sense of humour than mine commented it was a bit like 'owning your own weirdness', which I considered brilliant, as it summed up exactly how surreal being drink free felt at that point.

I already had my 100 days up on my wall chart, with a big red circle around October 27th. I really didn't think at the beginning I would last this long. Counting each and every day was ever so slowly becoming less relevant …

Chapter Four

I can count up to 100

Day 71
10 alternatives for alcohol

1. Give it away.
2. Paint your shed with it.
3. Pickle a body part in a jar with it.
4. Pour it down the sink.
5. Tie-dye a T-shirt with it.
6. Use it as lighter fluid for your barbeque.
7. Paint a picture with it.
8. Use it as ink to write with.
9. Leave it on the supermarket/store shelf.
10. Ignore it.

Friends were happy to contribute:

'Whenever I was not drinking previously, I used to freeze wine to use for cooking, then get desperate and defrost it! Plastic containers of wine, on top of the radiator, defrosting … I had people over for dinner last weekend and there was a third of a bottle of red left. Took me two days to throw it down the sink and I'm still disturbed that I don't find it easy to chuck out (the old mentality was that it would always get drunk the next day, the new line the devil comes up with is 'just in case you change your mind'). Freezer was too full to freeze it for cooking at a later date (another alternative use!) but have also found that replacing wine with extra stock in dishes makes little difference so haven't even been cooking with the stuff.'

Day 72
Living by my rules, not someone else's.

This weekend I had been mostly reviewing where I had come from and where I wanted to go next. I hated the fact that people who were stuck in a drinking mentality were in pain and wouldn't wish their traumas on my worst enemy, but at the same time thanked them for being brave enough to talk about it, because it reminded me of where I was 10 weeks ago and how much I never wanted those desperate, sometimes suicidal, emotions in my head ever again. I really hoped they managed to find a way to move forward.

One of the most significant moves forward for me had been the decision to make my own rules. It had been a revelation to me to realise that I had spent almost all of my life trying to please other people, and getting it hopelessly wrong, because the people I had tried to please kept changing the rules and, more importantly, were totally oblivious to how much pain I was in as a result of trying to please them. When I asked for help and admitted vulnerability they have turned their backs on me left me to it. When this first happened, and it has happened many times over my 47 years, I always blamed myself. But since packing in the drink and basically having what I believe now was some kind of breakdown, I had to step back, release, and stop trying to manage others' feelings about me. And guess what, I was free! I didn't worry about what they were thinking, feeling, needing, preferring, doing … I was thinking about me and my husband. It was making me well again.

We did our usual super stroll yesterday afternoon, eight or nine miles long the valley by the river Tyne, so beautiful in the sun, our little mutts rolling in bird shit (how idyllic) and the leaves all turning golden. I experienced a deep sense of peace. As a drinker I never had true peace.

I still had some sort of non-sleeping sickness, whatever the opposite of narcolepsy was, the symptoms of which were a) not sleeping b) not sleeping. I received much encouragement from online friends: 'Parallel paths … Something shifted this summer for me too. I feel free, free to be me and live the life I was meant to live, I think. Everything (and everyone) is being awarded its proper place and all perspectives are being aligned. Toxicity is slowly leaving this mind and body.'

Day 73
On the Persistence of Memory (Salvador Dali).

In discussions about symptoms, several people highlighted the strange dreams they had when going AF and how disturbing these could be. I had been plagued by vivid dreams since stopping drinking, and last night I dreamed an old watch I owned had melted and it was no longer possible to see the time on it. I looked up the meaning of this and the interpretation figured along the lines of what others have said to me about relaxing more:

'A clock or watch may simply represent the passage of time and indicate whether your dream refers to past, present, or future conditions. It may also show how your life is governed by the artificial routines created by organised society. Perhaps you should live a more carefree lifestyle that is less dependent on deadlines or "clock watching".'

Then, of course, there's Dali: 'The surrealist Artist Salvador Dali sometimes referred to his paintings as "hand-painted dream photographs" His famous picture, *The Persistence of Memory*, features melting clocks which are a reference to Dali's his lost and difficult childhood: the melting clocks are set on a beach near where he lived as a child.'

Funny old thing, the brain. It takes you to places you never knew existed when you slept, and yet it all made sense with a bit of thinking round the images. The gist seemed to be that funny dreams meant your brain was trying to tell you something that was buried deep down. Either way, it is a part of the experience that many people getting sober seem to share.

My most disturbing nightmares had been replaced by really vivid strange Dali-like dreams or drinking dreams (what a relief each time, to wake up and find I was still sober). It's funny because I had not dreamt much for years;

after a few glasses of wine I either didn't dream or couldn't remember. I was dreaming again and waking up remembering them; some odd, some strange, but all good because it was a sign that I was experiencing a better life.

Day 74

100 ways to distract yourself from needing a drink …

1. Bake a cake.
2. Have a bath: bubbles essential.
3. Plant some herbs for your windowsill.
4. Canoodle with your loved one (or by yourself, eh?).
5. Go for a long walk.
6. Do (more) housework.
7. Groom a pet/child.
8. Give yourself (or someone else) a false tan.
9. Pluck your eyebrows (or someone else's).
10. Exfoliate/body brush, shower, moisturise all over.
11. Build a flat pack.
12. Clear out your old clothes.
13. Read a book.
14. Listen to music.
15. Knit, sew, embroider, and/or crochet. Anything.
16. Go to the gym.
17. Plan your weekly food menus.
18. Make a nice lunch to take to work/out tomorrow.
19. Put on a face mask.
20. Defrost the freezer.
21. Make batches of healthy meals for the freezer (maybe wait till after it's refrosted).
22. Try doing your hair a different way.
23. Write your journal/diary.
24. Blog/post a discussion on Soberistas.
25. Paint a picture.
26. Write some poetry/a song.
27. Write a letter/email to a loved one.
28. Make your own clothes.
27. Call or go see a friend.
28. Do a workout/create a circuit training circuit.
29. Plan a holiday/adventure.

30. Get an exercise bike and knacker yourself out on it. Every night.
31. Eat biscuits.
32. Wash the car(s)
33. Clean out the rabbit(s)/ pets.
34. If unhappy where you are, apply for a new job.
35. Talk to your partner.
36. Set up your own blog/webpage.
37. Volunteer for a charity.
38. Do some CBT training so you can help others with the same problems.
39. Learn a new language.
40. Write a list of your good points.
41. Do facial exercises. Every night.
42. Make a model (did anyone else used to make Airfix models?)
43. Set up a train set and play with it.
44. Do out your shed, or get one and do it out as your den.
45. Dance in your dancing slippers.
46. Tell some jokes.
47. Give yourself a manicure/pedicure.
48. Practise putting on false eyelashes.
49. Practise new make-up.
50. Go window shopping and try on new clothes you wouldn't normally choose (don't have to buy them, or maybe save for later).
51. Try out new recipes.
52. Learn some DIY.
53. Play Scrabble (or another board game).
54. Get into video games.
55. Go on your Wii Fit.
56. Decide your new rules for life.
57. Practise positive statements about yourself.
58. Play tonsil tennis with another adult (maybe ask them first).

59. Join the Open University.
60. Write your book.
61. Practise sarcasm (but call it irony).
62. Tell someone your plans/dreams/aspirations.
63. Do a good deed.
64. Make a home-made present /card for someone.
65. Write a business plan for your money-making idea.
66. Then set up your new/part time/evening business.
67. Trade on eBay.
68. Self-publish on Kindle.
69. Play with your kids/dog/partner/friends/all.
70. Have a play wrestle.
71. Make up after an argument.
72. Get all the ironing done.
73. Devise a new mocktail.
74. Recycle some old furniture and sell it.
75. Make jewellery.
76. Sort out your finances.
77. File all that stuff that is sitting on your desk.
78. Have a massive clear out.
79. Get into Bonsai.
80. Cut/clip your partner's hair (ask them first).
81. Go to the pictures/watch a film.
82. Tell someone you love them.
83. Think.
84. Do yoga.
85. Clean the windows.
86. Set up your favourite programmes to record.
87. Make a batch of homemade muesli.
88. Go swimming.
89. Attend to hairy places (possibly before number 88).
90. Reorganise a room.
91. Learn self-hypnosis.
92. Make the appointment(s) you've been putting off.
93. Get an early night.
94. Make a hot chocolate with marshmallows and

squirty cream.
95. Go out and wheel the recycling bin around for the hell of it because it is so light and noiseless now.
96. Go for an eye test.
97. Get your MOT organised.
98. Repair something.
99. Train for a fun run.
100. Write yourself 100 things to do other than drinking.

Day 75
More better things to do than drinking.

I had an incident which upset me today. An alcoholic who had hardly managed a single session on one of my courses had to be told not to come any more, and got abusive and physically threatened me, telling me not to come to the centre tomorrow or else, all while drunk out of his skull. So tomorrow I have to be escorted into the building by a man and Reception instructed not to let anyone in unless I vet them first. My learners will have to be escorted out for their break-time cigarette and escorted back in again. I felt sorry for this person and also very, very sad.

Anyway. On to some daftness. Instead of having a drink:

101. Change all the names on your phone so everyone has a nickname.
102. Make brownies and cupcakes and give them away tomorrow.
103. Learn how to tile and redo your bathroom.
104. Make a swear box.
105. Polish your halo.

Bonus:

106. Book a week in a cottage over Christmas without discussing it with your husband first …

Day 76
Christmas decision time.

This year had been a time of massive changes, especially since going AF.

I booked a little cottage in the Lake District for a week over Christmas. It was a few minutes from the beach, with views of the Solway Firth, not much happening except the Irish Sea, wind, rain, fresh air, sand, and pebbles. Two border terriers and a husband and some unashamed self-indulgence. Husband was pretty surprised by the news that we were going there, but took it well. The cottage was a little stone place with thick walls and low ceilings. I was in love.

On another note: I HATE TURKEY (damn that felt good).

Sorry to any turkeys reading this, nothing personal, but you are boring and tasteless. Come to think, of it there are a few humans like that and all. Our dinner of choice was roast beef sandwiches, plus roast potatoes, with excellent bread buns, and plenty of gravy to dip with. Who cared what the rest of the world was having; I could be a sober rebel and revel!

People online were also considering how to deal with Christmas: 'Really good idea to start thinking about how to do it at Christmas now. When the evenings are getting dark, and the pubs have those boards outside offering mulled wine – it is a very seductive thing – there's a strong persuasion to get back into drinking. However, what happens after that? How many more drinkies go down, and then what about the next day? I too am regarding Christmas with some apprehension, because the red wine flows like water at my parents' on Boxing Day. Will just have to remember 'No thanks, I don't drink, no thanks, I don't drink, no thanks, I don't drink.'

Christmas has started playing on my mind a bit. I knew

for many the challenge of Christmas seemed huge without a drink and it felt great to have a plan in place. I reminded myself how distinctly flat I felt after last Christmas and saying 'it all went in a bit of a blur really' (absolute blur – I was pissed or hungover for most of it). I was looking forward to remembering everything this year.

Day 77
Offer hope and friendship, rather than a drink.

A dear lady on Soberistas, who was sprucing up her sewing room, inspired me to make some changes in our own home. Our two spare bedrooms were now separate dens/offices for me and husband, so he could be a neat freak in his space and I could spread my stuff out in mine. Having a separate den was quite liberating and inspiring, even generating a feeling of reincarnation. It was amazing how good it felt to just move stuff around and create some personal space – much as I loved the person I was getting space from.

Highs and lows seem to be how recovery took me, still. One minute I was feeling full of the joys and the next I was stressed to fuck again, wondering what could go wrong, even when nothing was actually going wrong. That feeling of 'oh we're all going to hell' when to be honest, if I sat myself down and gave myself a proper talking too, life was pretty much exactly the same as it was a couple of hours ago when nothing at all was awry. There was no predicting when these moods would take me. I was even wondering if I was starting the menopause, it was that bad.

Dealing with these regular and often extreme fluctuations in moods had been one of the trickiest parts of recovery, hormones or not. I think what was assumed by me was that I have had this depression/anxiety disorder for many, many years, because of drinking. Maybe, though, there was no chicken and egg (I often wondered if I drank because I was depressed or was depressed because I drank), but in fact two different issues going on. Maybe the drink was incidental to a much deeper problem. I found I was reincarnated as a sober but a bit depressed person. I took the anti ds I was on originally to offset the effects of quitting drinking, but I now questioned if there more to the different things going on in my brain than simply getting over an addiction. Maybe the depression I experienced as a child and teen, before I started drinking, never really went away.

The new den and the growing self-awareness ran hand in hand.

Day 78
The revolutionary AF effect.

I ordered new walking boots for me and OH as we were going quite a few miles at the weekends. We both felt so much better for these long walks and looked forward to the peace and quiet they brought us.

I had a homeless man on my current course; he was hoping to get a flat, but in the meantime I and the learners brought in bread and ham and biscuits to take home. It broke my heart to see a sixty-year-old man in that position. The good news is he hasn't had a drink in two weeks and I got one of the other learners to take him to the local opticians for an eye test as he could barely see. There were always people so much worse off, so my feeling was we have a responsibility to look after ourselves properly by not drinking, so that we could be in a position to help others. That sounds so sanctimonious, but it was one of the motivations I used to stay AF. I could not be there for people if I was in a state myself.

I had another learner tell me that since we had a group chat about alcohol and I mentioned the link with breast cancer she came to tell me she had cut right back, and this lady was known in the area (everyone knew everyone around Durham, it seemed) for liking a drink.

So not trying to blow my own trumpet but I was really proud that in small ways my own decision to get clean has had small effects on other people. *Viva la revolución!*

Day 79
What would you say to your drunk self?

I had been tut-tutting at programmes on the telly like *Bouncers*, some of which was filmed in my part of the world, but the truth of the matter was that I had been just as shitfaced and outrageous on many occasions. People may say, 'Well you can move on from that now,' but personally I thought it did me no harm at all to remember How It Used To Be.

So I was in my late teens, early twenties and I saw myself coming into a bar with a big group of friends, many of whom I had met that night through friends of friends of friends and would never see again. But we were all best buddies. I was screaming with laughter at something hilarious I had just heard, but my mood changed like wildfire when someone accidentally bumped my drink and it spilt down my top. Even though they were apologetic I still threw my weight around (four more stone of it than now) just so they knew that I was so much better than them and they did right to be apprehensive of me. I pushed in to get to the bar because my drink was finished and I had to have another one straightaway or I would feel like I was missing out, and while on the way there flirted with a few strangers, mentally congratulating myself on wearing the gear I bought for the occasion of getting drunk and the money I spent on make-up because some other drunken unimportant arseholes noticed me enough to bother to respond to my idiotic comments.

Fast forward a decade and I was out in an expensive wine bar in town and I saw myself with my first husband, having had a few wines while getting ready and by eight o'clock had had enough to sink the *Titanic* and certainly I was sinking fast. I repeated myself a lot and talked general bollocks, entertaining strangers with amusing stories of our horrible marriage and listened totally rapt to while they talked drunken bollocks, while my husband sat increasingly angry and bemused, wondering how soon we were to go home because I could not walk or talk any more. Then I peered through the curtains at myself at home, watching the drunken row that thank God the neighbours did not hear because our cottage was detached, and I watched him raise his hand to me to shut me the fuck up, and I was on the floor, winded, and he stepped over me to go to bed, shutting the door behind him and leaving me, heaving, on the floor, alone and cold and pissed and wishing I was dead.

Trot forward another five years and I was waiting for my internet date to pick me up from my singleton house, a house bought with a minimum deposit from the meagre proceeds of my divorce. Not caring we hardly knew each other, I had never been to his home, and I only had his mobile phone number as ID. Many years of drinking made me reckless, although I thought of it as carefree and empowered at the time. No one could hurt me, neither emotionally or physically. I was perfectly willing to inflict violence on or damage the property of anyone that tried, such was the damage done to my mental health by the Drink Demon by then.

I had already had a drink or two while getting ready as was my established habit in my house, drinking alone nightly, whether I was going out later or staying in with the soaps, loud rock music pumping me up, my bloated face in the mirror telling me I looked great, despite the mid-thirties cigarettes and alcohol-generated lines starting to appear around my nose, mouth, and eyes, the drink flushing my cheeks a little too much, my belly a little too distended from red wine and too much junk food, but hidden by an expensive designer wrap top. Throw some money at it and made it go away, all very straightforward from my position of wine-induced superiority.

He was a respectable enough guy, a community mental

health worker as it happened, and I judged him trustworthy. Even though he told me he was recently separated from his wife and had two small kids, I was confident the marriage was over. I chose to believe what I wanted to believe. I took him to a barbeque of a teacher friend who was taking early retirement after many years, selling the family home and going off travelling with her hubby in a campervan, now her children were all grown up. The guests all had a perfectly fun night as I remember; it was fine, warm evening in May. Some got a little tipsy, but I got so blasted my date had to carry me to my car and drive my vehicle home (I had offered to drive there, in the vain hope this tactic would ensure I stayed off too much booze). We didn't say much that I could remember on the way home, but I smelt his disappointment and embarrassment like a petrol-soaked rag.

He carried me into the house and I remembered annoying him by being awkward about going up to the bedroom and having a mini wrestle in the hall which eventually made him half drag me, half kick me up the stairs, saying he wanted to make sure I got safely to bed. In my half dead state he pushed me face forward onto the bed, removed the lower half of my clothes, and I felt a sharp stabbing pain in my behind as he forced himself on me, and then I was unconscious.

When I came to, some hours later, the sun was highlighting up my half-dressed body through open curtains, the pigeons were cooing in their usual irritating way, traffic noise as normal. I stood up and immediately pissed myself, urine and blood mixing down my leg, and all I could think was, I just had these floorboards polished. So I cleaned myself up, very sore, and texted this 'man', 'Why did you do that to me?' but I never saw or heard from him again.

I went to work as normal on the Monday, but I didn't hear a single word any child or adult said to me, I just nodded and smiled. I learned to do that a lot. I switched off from nearly everything and everyone, apart from the Drink Demon.

So I said to myself seven years on from that, nothing had really changed, except that I was a bit older and looked a bit more ridiculous when drunk, and people humoured me a bit more, and I was bit more skint and a bit more depressed and a bit more unstable. I answered, well, clever arse, stuff you, because actually now I only drank a few glasses a week; OK they might be big glasses, but I still held down a job, didn't I? I was not like an alcoholic, I didn't do stuff that alcoholics did. Oh yes, my friend, I said to myself, you weren't yet sitting a park bench with a can of Carling like the gentlemen and ladies of the road, quite right. But you were stuck, my friend, and quietly desperate, and quietly sad that you have fucked up or been fucked up, over and over again. You have lived a life of quiet desperation, waiting for that ultimate risky, hazardous, and life-threatening action that would finish you and send you across to that bench, or to that hospital bed, or to that wheelchair, or to those courts, or to that hole in the ground. Your luck is running out.

So I took that woman and shook her and told her enough was enough. And she agreed. And now was where we were.

Day 80
Being proactive after so many years of reactive.

God, sometimes don't you feel like you've been on the planet such a long time? Looking back on stuff, I was constantly jolted by how many years ago things happened, and yet they still cut like a knife if I ever let them. But I was learning to stick a big red stop sign up in my brain when painful things tried to haunt me again, and pushed them back into their rightful place, which was in the memory bin.

So there was a new thing going on in the flat, which was deciding to stop bad things happening before they happened, rather than allowing them to happen and then thrashing about in a panic trying to sort out the problem. This included:

- Thinking about what I actually want to happen and doing something about it, rather than dwelling on what I fear might happen and sitting like a rabbit in the headlights waiting for it to become a self-fulfilling prophesy.
- Not allowing negative people/situations to interfere with my recovery.
- Not being ashamed of being reflective and considerate towards myself.
- Getting into the habit of replacing negative mental statements/thinking with positive ones.
- Being OK about avoiding social/recreational events (and therefore certain people) which now bore me witless or are a complete chore.
- Being happy in my own company while sober.
- Making allowances for people who have their own shit going on and not seeing it as a personal slight if they appear to take it out on me.

I think these new organization resolutions were rooted

in my recent dreams, where I was forever missing a plane, not having my passport or tickets, going to the wrong classroom to teach, or generally just not being able to get where I wanted on time. So it was definitely time to start planning rather than just waiting for what was round the corner and hoping for the best. I wanted to lose some more weight, finally see off the Drink Demon and the Sugar Monster, to be better organised at work, to have the house cleaner, and to be better with money – all of which I had previously worried about but done nothing to change until things were unbearable. But packing in drinking and being proactive taught me that I had more power over my life than I thought. It was possible to take these new skills of self-control and self-knowledge and use them in so many other areas of life, or as a friend called them, 'transferable skills.'

Day 81
Thinking of taking a drink? Craving a cheeky one?

What do you actually know about the alcohol in your Chablis/Prosecco/Barolo? Here's the sciency stuff.

Ethanol, known by most as alcohol, is the principal psychoactive constituent in alcoholic beverages, with depressant effects on the central nervous system. It has a complex mode of action and affects multiple systems in the brain, most notably increasing the activity of GABA receptors. Through positive allosteric modulation, it enhances the activity of naturally produced GABA. Other psychoactives such as benzodiazepines and barbiturates exert their effects by binding to the same receptor complex, thus have similar CNS depressant effects.

Still feel like a good glass of Chardonnay?

Day 82
10 better things to spend £5.99 on than Pinot.

1. A present for someone.
2. Donate £5.99 to charity.
3. Spend £5.99 on cleaning products and muck out the house.
4. Some lovely bath products for a decadent old soak.
5. A takeaway pizza (and eat the lot yourself).
6. A box of choccies.
7. Some seeds or a plant for your garden. These are great to remind you as they grow of how far you've come since becoming AF.
8. A book, magazine, or DVD you have wanted for ages.
9. Stick it in your piggy bank towards something bigger.
10. Something nice for your children, partner, or pet.

Thoughts from a few friends of mine revealed more truths about just how much you can save by going AF:

'2 weeks' wine money is enough for me to go for a pamper/salon day. Now that I'm AF, I go twice a month.'

'I've shocked myself with how much I've saved by cutting out those £5.99s. I've treated myself to a 3-month gym pass, to see me through Christmas instead. Much healthier. ☺'

I knocked back several invites because I just could not face watching people get drunk. But if I could not get out of it and really had to go (did I REALLY have to go?) then I considered the options:

- Stay for the minimum time that is polite (borderline

people pleasing).

• Leave AS SOON AS the Drink Demon (or any other unpleasant character) started to play with my mind.

• Be up front about not drinking. It didn't matter what white lie I told; my motivation was none of their business. I didn't have to justify a damn thing).

• Stand up for myself if someone called me boring, or hinted I was not one of the team. I prepared the responses in advance.

• Plan what I would drink and stick to it so I wasn't caught out by indecision.

• Ask my partner or a friend for support so they could stick up for me too, and help if I panicked.

• Look my absolute best.

• Most of all be proud and remember I had friends who would always support me.

• Remember I didn't play the Drink Demon's games any more.

• Covertly replace any alcoholic drinks served to me with non-alcoholic ones.

On a recent night out with the girls I got my own drinks in – a Monster energy drink with loads of ice – and the barman asked if I wanted vodka, and the look on his face when I said no, ha, It cost me just £1.09, whereas the others were buying bottles of Prosecco (yes, each) at nearly £15 quid a time, and drinking them in not much less time than I had my modest Monster. I have been there, done that, got the video, burnt the T-shirt.

Day 83
Could be worse. You could have auto-brewery syndrome.

I was sitting watching my local news agog at the item on a poor chap who had a something called 'auto brewery syndrome', where any carbs he ate fermented in his gut and turned to alcohol. If this gentleman ate too many carbs, he could end up with alcohol poisoning. Imagine not even being able to have any carbs at all? There are always people worse off than ourselves.

I was doing something newly positive every day, and I really hoped there were people out there also doing this in order to cut the drink out once and for all. I was finding a proactive approach took my mind off drinking and planning activities and gave me something positive to think about.

I was doing my usual stretching out like a starfish on the bed when I came in, when I heard some suspicious chewing. One of them had hold of one of my £40 Next ankle boots, and had chewed through the zip and was busy with the toe area. So instead of shouting and remaining irritable with my mutt long after he had forgotten what it was he had done, thereby rendering the exercise pointless, I decided to be positive about this distressing experience and simply order myself a new pair of boots. Happy Christmas.

Day 84
Giving my body a present.

I would never be complacent about alcohol and was well aware that the addiction could sneak up on you when you least expect it. I was never that far from saying, 'Sod it', and if I looked deep down into myself. I suspect I will always have that in me. The key is to be mindful and to see addiction for what it is: not your personality or who you are, but an illness that needed to be treated as such. Just as people were prone to backache or flu, it could come back and needed to be dealt with using practical and logical measures.

Having reached a reasonably comfortable (dare I say smug) point of nearly 3 months (OMG), I was feeling far more positive about the possibility of the above. I found myself thinking about what else I did to my poor ageing body and the biggies which affected my mood, weight, bank balance, and so on just like alcohol used to do; caffeine and sugar. I knew I could polish things up a bit more in this little insular life I lead if I quit these and started nourishing myself properly.

The possibility of giving up caffeine/sugar meant I could manage my depression a bit more easily than just swallowing pills. I wanted to come off these anti ds and I suspected if I could modify my diet/intake of stimulants I would be able to look at this as a way forward for the new year. I can't wait!

Day 85
A face like a twice-dropped pie.

I did seem to have replaced alcohol with eating total crap and was very unhappy with myself.

I had begun to treat sugar just like alcohol; I had no self-control and was always going too far. I would buy a family-sized cheesecake and gobble the lot before it even got to the fridge. I would buy a four-pack of Wispa Golds and munch through them in less than an hour. Chocolate cookies didn't stand a chance; the whole packet would be gone while I unpacked the shopping. It was actually scaring me how much I was not in control of this. I knew it wasn't as big a deal as an alcohol addiction, but having come so far, I couldn't stand the feeling of not being in control of what I put in my mouth.

I had a feeling the only way I could master this was by applying the same logic as I applied to drinking and plan it the same way. Bye-bye sugar, hello new running shoes (hopefully the dogs won't chew these too).

I used to run as a kid and did a few half marathons; it was a thing I loved that I had forgotten I loved. I decided the weekend would be a great time to try the 'Couch to 5K' app on my phone – a nine week app which gets you from total beginner to able to run a 5K.

Day 86
A happy wife (or happy significant other) makes for a better life.

Good things happened today.

It was Friday and that would normally fill me with a certain amount of gloom because I missed the usual celebratory drinks, but for the first Friday since becoming AF I didn't have these cravings at all! I was going whole daytimes without thinking about drink, and when a drink thought came into my head it was more of a surprise than anything else.

The company I worked for was moving me out of the tiny rooms I trained in for one particular course and into somewhere bigger and better.

OH provided me with takeaway pizza and AF ginger ale this evening, which he paid for out of his wages as he has obtained work, albeit temporarily, but it was money coming in after a desperate period. He was also happily tired and looking forward to the football on the telly as a working man. He also said a happy wife makes for a better life, which to me is the ultimate wisdom.

So there was a fair bit of smuggy in the nest this evening.

Day 87
Honesty is a gift to those who deserve it.

I've had a few more thoughts recently about something which had once really worried me, namely what to tell others about the decision to become AF.

This is understandable if you are anxious about what other people think and don't want them to be upset, or for them to know there is a problem.

One of the hardest lessons I had to learn was that what other people need to know was actually based what I decided they needed to know. I was not being deceitful or letting people down if I did not tell them exactly what was on my mind. In some cases, I was doing them a favour and protecting them so they didn't have to dwell on my problems. In some cases I simply didn't know or like them enough to tell them the truth about my AF because frankly it was none of their business. In some cases I got a perverse and satisfying pleasure from not telling them the real reasons for my decision to look after myself properly from now on. In some cases I didn't like them enough to want them to know the secret of how wonderful I was feeling.

I could honestly say that my true feelings and reasons about why I didn't drink were only ever discussed with a few people, either anonymously on forums or private messaging with my new AF friends, and with my OH. That was my choice and I was comfortable with it. I told a range of people elsewhere a range of information about not drinking, depending on my mood or need for privacy or my pure obstinacy.

A friend of mine commented on keeping your own counsel: 'I told my boss last week and I really regret it! I know what other people think of you is their business but it bothers me that he now thinks I'm a bit of a bore. Lesson learnt methinks! Going to think twice, next time, before sharing my AF status, with anyone. Isn't it funny (as in peculiar) that some people think less of us for not drinking? It is the best decision I ever made, the best 20 months of my life and my gift to my baby boys. And yet it still bothers me what people think.'

Day 88
What is your gift to others?

A super friend really affected me with a comment she made about her sobriety being her gift to her children, and I so admired her for this brave and hugely significant way of looking at being AF. Thanks to her, for putting certain things in perspective.

I did the pub and an Indian meal after last night – the kind of normal stuff that in the past would have seen me preloading with wine from about 5 p.m. As I had my getting ready drink I wouldn't think about the fact that my OH was not happy about me going out half cut, and the fact that he would have to bring me home early 9 times out of 10 because I was beyond conversation, or talking too much to complete strangers and basically ignoring him. My gift to him was my sobriety and it changed our relationship so much that I knew it was the best pressie I could give him. He told me last night that I was no longer grumpy and argumentative, that my horrendous PMS cycle was no longer as pronounced, and that I was glowing physically.

Yesterday I gave myself a gift by not having any chocolate. I cannot remember when I last did a day without chocolate. I turned down chocolate offered by OH, who now knows not to do that now (poor bloke, he never knew what was coming next), I left the little wrapped chocolate I found on the pub table and I turned down the After Eight mints concluding our meal out. Three times I would have had it.

I made myself stay busy and hardly had a minute on the sofa, which was where most of the chocolate/wine habit took place. I actually lost some of my appetite which was weird, but I knew if I ate a lot of sugar it just made me want to eat more and more of everything.

Day 89
What have the Drink Demon and an allotment got in common?

Took my OH into town this morning and subjected him to open wallet surgery, poor lad was no doubt glad of some peace this afternoon when I went outside into my allotment to potter. He called me Trixie, which was short for Beatrix Potter, because of my love of pottering about. I could waste hours pottering without actually getting anything of any consequence done, but at least I was no longer doing it with a can or a glass at my side, or sneaky tabs in my pocket.

I literally kicked, raked, dug, battered with the back of the spade, and stamped the shit out of the soil I needed to shift from one place to another in order to create a raised area for sitting out in next year (the neighbours were arranging to have me committed, no doubt).

I inflicted similar treatment, mentally, on the Drink Demon and it was a quivering wreck, loitering in the corner. I moved it from one area of my brain to a more convenient and comfortable area, like the soil in my veggie patch. I rubbed earth all over its face and mine and then laughed about it maniacally. It didn't dare even speak. It hadn't yet completely effed off, but I was working on that. Destroy what destroys you. I could thoroughly recommend pottering and both real and symbolic earth moving for straightening one's thoughts.

Day 90
How people pleasing affects your health.

I now saw I was not alone in continuing to drink so I kept others happy. That meant saying yes to a drink when I really wanted to say no, it meant trying to give up a thousand times and only managing a few days before social pressures got me yet again, and it meant putting my deepest needs on the back burner for the sake of fitting in.

People pleasing had been the bane of my life for decades. I can remember doing things to try and fit in and get approval since I was small child, into teenage years, as a young adult, and then into my thirties trying to numb out because I felt such a failure for putting myself to one side all that time. Drink was an enabler, allowing me to switch off from myself and giving me a focus/excuse for the times when other people's needs were more important than mine.

I didn't have drinking buddies any more. It was a heavy price in some respects but it was also the most liberating experience of my entire life because I was compromising for no one. I was who I was and the new possibilities were endless. All the extra thinking time and the pleasure of making decisions to suit me. Selfish? No more selfish than people around us who tried to force their wishes on us and most of the time succeeded when we were made vulnerable by alcohol. Shift the alcohol from your life and you could start shifting the people pleasing too. And some of the people.

Day 91
Not taking any crap.

I'm so pleased to report I was on chocolate free day 5, and this was a major event in my little life, as I could honestly not remember going a day without chocolate or a related sweet snack, pretty much ever. I knew most people experienced massive sugar cravings as part of the withdrawal, but I wanted to offer hope to those currently struggling with this secondary battle. I was finding that it most definitely did calm itself down. A few weeks ago I would never have believed it, as I reckoned sweet crap was part of my life for ever. But this fight with cravings and slowly winning was another string to my strengthening bow.

I had a row with OH last night over the state of the house – now he was working he hadn't time to do all the housework as he did before and I haven't stepped up. I shouted at him about it but actually I needed to review this. I was sorry. So today I was having the day off and I was going to blitz the place so that all the piles of crap were dispersed (lovely image) and he could feel a bit more comfortable when he got in.

Day 92
The Real Causes of Compulsive Drinking?

I have cleaned more of our modest flat than I have ever cleaned in my entire life. You may think I'm joking, but the back yard is full if crap to take to the tip tomorrow.

In between cleaning and shifting things around I have been reading about my continuing symptoms of alcohol/food cravings. Thanks to the website weightandwellness.com from where I got great advice and have written/edited the following using their content:

Was it a matter of chemistry?

The psychological approach to correcting obsessive drinking suggests that I should identify my feelings before I take the first drink. Am I lonely, sad, happy, or all of the above? Once I take the first drink, I am on the fast track to a binge.

People's drink struggles are repeated over and over. People are frustrated with the answers they have been given from family members, friends, and even professionals. Nothing has helped this debilitating, guilt-ridden behaviour that chokes away self-esteem.

The true solution to compulsive overeating and drinking (the two are frequently linked compulsions – certainly for me) comes from understanding the biochemistry of your cravings. An acceptance of your own personal biochemistry is critical. Once you take on personal responsibility for your biochemistry, you take charge of your food cravings and compulsive drinking.

Out of control blood sugar

Research has confirmed many people simply cannot drink alcohol and cannot eat sugar and grains without it leading to out-of-control behaviour. You can check this out for yourself. Examine the sensitive nature of your own blood sugar (the highs and lows); the cravings created and the physical, emotional, and mental response you have to both high and low blood sugar. What happens to your blood sugar when you eat a high carbohydrate diet or down a high sugar bottle of wine?

It doesn't matter which processed carbohydrate food or drink you choose, carbohydrates break down into sugar (glucose) in your body and go into your blood. Unbalanced blood sugar levels are a major cause of carbohydrate cravings. Hence the hangover cravings.

Because your blood cannot tolerate too much sugar, your body naturally produces the hormone insulin that takes sugar from the blood and deposits it into the cells. When you eat a high carbohydrate meal or drink more than the recommended units of alcohol, your blood sugar can rise to a dangerous level. Large doses of insulin rush to the scene and clear out the sugar. As a result of clearing, the opposite state occurs, called low blood sugar.

You may be familiar with feeling low blood sugar – being tired, irritable, or even shaky. To bring blood sugar back up, your body sends your brain a chemical message saying, 'I need sugar, eat sugar (or drink sugar in the form of wine etc.)' Hence you crave pop/soda, bread, brownies, pasta, or anything with sugar … like booze. In effect, your booze cravings are a biochemical response to low blood sugar. Cravings are not a lack of will power!

The sweet side of alcohol addiction

If you have traded an alcohol addiction (sugar) for a sweet thing addiction (sugar), you have gained little more than a lessened risk for the same illnesses that too much sugar can bring on.

Biochemically, sugar and alcohol are the same thing.

When you take in large amounts of sugar it sends your blood sugar high and releases a feel-good neurotransmitter called serotonin. The alcohol and the sweet thing both send your blood sugar high, but the alcohol is able to spike your blood sugar twice as fast. So if you have stopped taking in alcohol and replaced it with high sugar eating/drinking, you are setting yourself up for a relapse.

If you are ready to put an end to this cycle, you need to be eating balanced meals every three to four hours and taking some amino acids to help rebuild and heal your brain chemistry. Balanced meals should consist of protein, fat, and carbohydrates. For healthy protein, eat chicken, fish, beef, cheese, and steak. For fat, choose butter, olive oil, raw nuts, and cream cheese. For carbohydrates, choose fruits and lots of veggies.

Helping out the brain

For some people, compulsive drinking is related to deficiencies in neurotransmitters. If you lack serotonin, dopamine, or one of the other essential chemical communicators in your brain, the resulting behaviour is cravings for carbohydrates, especially sugar.

Antibiotics and sugar cravings

Cravings and lack of control have a biochemical connection to the unhealthy condition of the intestinal tract. Have you noticed that you have more sugar cravings after a round of antibiotic treatment? Rebalancing your gut with probiotics can tame those cravings before they take over.

So, to stop the craving for alcohol which your body is seeing as a way of obtaining sugar … kill the sugar and you kill the Drink Demon and tame the Sugar Monster at the same time.

I realised that if we looked at this sweet craving thing from a science point of view and separated it from the emotions (which still needed to be dealt with) the cravings became easier to deal with. If you get the cravings, have something healthy to eat, and start training your brain to despise sugar. But if like me you want to be free of your body telling you what to do and be in control of your reactions, then the chemical reaction of sugar in the body needed to be understood and dealt with.

Day 93
Wear your AF badge of honour with pride.

Well done to everyone celebrating any kind of AF, whether it is five minutes, five hours, five days …

I was proud to say on October 27th I would have lived 100 days completely AF, and have learned a lot of things about myself on the way that I really should have cottoned on to a long time ago, but was too busy examining the bottom of a glass. I was doing months now and counted the 19th of every month as a special day. I would probably always count this, even as the days and weeks turned into years.

As well as everyone else who was trying their best, I was so proud to be in the same company online as people who had gone a lot longer than me AF – they kept me going and made me want to prove I could do it too. There were times when being a competitive pain in the ass was a good thing, because turning that energy towards something positive rather than to being a better drinker than everyone else was actually making me into a better person. Spending time giving to other people, in no matter how minute a way, made me feel like I was not the disappointing, career-screwing, money-throwing, attitude-stinking waste of space some people thought I was; the girl (not the woman) with pure brass neck to think she could ever write or be anything of any consequence. I actually felt worth something and my online friends gave me that without even realising they did it.

So the next time you questioned whether you should dare write a blog or comment on one, or make yourself known to someone, or befriend someone you admire or want to help, the next time you questioned if you should, then go right ahead, because you would be making someone out there feel very special with only a tiny few words. You too should be wearing your AF badge of honour, no matter how long it has been.

Day 94
What in the name of God's flip flops is going on?

Alcohol seemed to be everywhere today. I got one set of train tickets earlier for the London meeting of online friends and in with them was a £40 money-off token for a case of wine. We went to the pictures tonight and saw Stallone in *The Escape Plan*, and at the kiosks you could buy glasses of wine and bottles of lager to take in with you, but sadly no coffee or tea.

I watched an episode of *Saturday Kitchen* I had recorded and they were sitting round drinking expensive wine at ten in the morning, having orgasms over the fruity undertones. Then there were adverts for Southern Comfort, Guinness, and Carling on ITV before lunch.

Corrie and *Eastenders* were on catch-up and in practically every scene someone had a glass of alcohol in their hand. Later when I went to the corner shop, the entire length of one wall of the shop was devoted to drink.

I could go on.

Day 95
Serene Swan Sunday.

Sweeping majestically across the lake of life, gazing down at the weeds and thinking, I'm going to eat you in a minute pal …

Reaching 100 days was so close, I could taste it, like the swans reaching out for the weeds. I had no swan pretentions, but it was lovely to feel calm and peaceful about the world, and just glide a bit. It was like coming in to land with wings spread wide and beady eyes on the prize; a healthy and productive future.

Day 96
Decluttering.

My physical decluttering of last week had started off mental decluttering, too. I was looking at pictures of my wedding and other happy events and wanting to make an album to remind myself of the good times, but in so many I could see I'd been drinking, and so many were of me looking overweight and out of shape. So I was not going to do that. Today's thing was to declutter my photos physically and in my head so the ones where I am half pissed, completely pissed, and looking stodgy podgy were out of my life. I was making a new mental and physical photo album that I actually looked at with pride and optimism for the future.

I was pleased to say I had not missed chocolate or crisps after the first few days and had cut down on white flour massively, all of which was helping, and small steps would do it. I knew some people say, well what on earth will you have to look forward to you crazy cow, but for me the thing to look forward to was being fit and well physically and mentally.

You can't beat a bit of decluttering. Nothing makes me happier than throwing lots of old crap out of the attic that I have kept just in case. But decluttering the old head space is a bit harder. We do accumulate a bit of rubbish up there!

Day 97
Does anyone know anything about Ang B?

'Cos she's bang out of order as far as I'm concerned!

Sorry.

That terrible joke was about as exciting as my Friday nights felt; thought it must be the weather and a sore neck making me feel a bit low, even though it was not different to any of the 13 other AF Friday nights I have had. I didn't want a drink, because I was used to following through as it were, making myself rehearse what happened after the first sip, the first glass, the first bottle … it was always the same unpleasant scenario. So by the time I thought through what happened when I took a drink, every single time, I went off the idea.

Day 98
Sand Dunes.

Climbing sand dunes today at our local beach, I realised I have been at the bottom of a metaphorical dune for quite a long time. I could have chosen to stay at the bottom of it and admire the view. The dunes are after all pretty spectacular, when viewed from the beach.

At the top of the dunes, I discovered that not only could I still see the beach, I could also see the wide expanse of the North Sea, with little white boats out and about, enjoying the sunshine, and all around me the rugged countryside, for miles and miles. Little dots of people in the distance. What a brilliant feeling; it was worth getting out of puff to get to the top and to experience success.

While walking the coastal path, my other half and I talked about how some people chose football teams to support simply because they were successful, yet he seemed 'addicted' to a team which continually failed. The thing is though, they never gave up, although he might disagree!

He felt he didn't have a choice; he chose this team and would stay loyal to them no matter what. He hoped they would get to the top of their particular sporting dune and be able to see more sea, more countryside, more possibilities. Didn't stop him cursing them though. We all had hill to climb, a tricky team to support, our own deep-rooted issues and insecurities to master – at least, the majority of us. It was whether we chose to keep climbing, or kicking the fecking ball, that counted.

I had been pretty wrung out this last 98 days with my own doings. But I had no choice but to carry on, or I would always be at the bottom of my own particular dune. Not nice to loiter there long term, when the view from the top was so spectacular.

Day 99

99 problems but the booze ain't one!

It had been a tricky 99 days and I still felt raw about leaving alcohol behind forever, but life was so short and it was so important to think about the good stuff, or else the bad stuff threatened to drag me down to where I was. I was still taking anti-depressants and dealing with anxiety. I was sad to get a letter from the mental health people saying there was a huge waiting list for a counsellor, so possibly that was not as bright a star as I thought. I would join the list however and wait in hope, like so many others needing someone to talk to.

But it wasn't all bad; it never was. I was so grateful that this journey generated many new friends, both in the cyber world and by actually meeting up. I spent a long time withdrawn from people in general. I walked away from friends who were still drinking and from a social life where all that really happened was the pub, house parties, and more drinking excuses. Suddenly events that seemed fabulous because drink was the main thing on the menu became not so clever. I worried it was a lack in me that I could not do 'old' stuff anymore, that my tolerance level for drinking environments had gone right down. I shied away from social stuff still, and felt fear, no other word for it, even when going out for a simple meal. I got proper agoraphobic sensations which made me anxious and shrivelled.

People told me it took guts to write everything down and I was proud of myself for doing it. I still had a sense that not everyone was pleased for us sober bloggers putting ourselves out there, exposing our lives and feelings, trying to make sense of this new life. Many people saw our viewpoints as threats, our humour as arrogant, our opinions as ridiculous. I was so proud to be a part of a movement for change. I didn't expect to be liked, but I did want my boundaries respected and to respect others' boundaries.

Day 100
Reflections on 100 days.

I got there! The most amazing feeling and one I will remember forever. I thrashed about and moaned and whooped and generally made a noise, cried and huffed and puffed, laughed, sighed, been disappointed and elated, frustrated and relieved … every emotion I can think of has happened, come and gone, and replaced the numbness that was being a drinker. I welcomed all of these confusing and liberating feelings, because they were real, and they were showing me that there was actually a person in there who was worth something.

Triple digits seemed so significant, because it meant that the first struggle was over, and there was a happy, healthy future to look forward to.

Folk who get sober and stay that way are justifiably proud of their achievement and anything which helps to develop that community spirit is surely no bad thing. Hence the blogging madly, obsessively, continually. Even if I felt the blogging urge was less compulsive these days, I still held it responsible for my sobriety.

From the massively important to the frivolous, I loved the way bloggers provided news about the growing community interest, 'sobriety', and in doing so, showed people that living without drinking to excess was perfectly possible. I loved being part of that movement, and still do.

Interaction is a crucial part of developing a sober community, which is why blogging is so valuable, by people from all walks of life, no matter how much they have been/are drinking. The last thing sobriety needs is to sound dull, and as many different people writing about it as possible is a key outcome for helping others quit dependent drinking. No matter what their political views, social situation, or personal standpoints, it is great to hear others' take on sober life. I love the fact that in the blogs I read there is no rigid 'party line' – simply a desire to assist as many people as possible find the right recovery route for them as individuals. Participation in the debate is healthy.

What exactly is a sober community? We have diverse religious, ethnic, and socio-economic backgrounds, live in different parts of the world, and yet we have the issue of how to overcome alcohol addiction to unite us. An issue based community is completely apt and relevant for modern life and together we can play an increasingly important role in influencing policy makers.

Many of us feel alone in trying to overcome addiction to alcohol, but unified by a common strand we can overcome differences potentially generated by demographic, geography, tastes, lifestyle preferences, and a whole raft of others. We can open up avenues to walk together which will empower us all as a group, rather than trying to tackle the issues alone, as well as providing opportunities to cherish and nurture the emerging heroes who work on our behalf.

The internet provides a future for social communication no matter where in the world we are. The things that really matter to a community of sober people can be explored, developed, pursued. New information can be disseminated in seconds and impact directly on the lives of people who need support. Sometimes the internet is the only outlet people have to meet others in the same situation.

The great thing about being AF is that you started to consider new possibilities and the risk-taking behaviour was transformed from self-harming to positive action which benefited both yourself and other people. The time, money, and energy I used to expend in managing (barely) my drinking and occasionally having to do damage limitation were now spent in doing stuff that made me and my partner happier people. These may be things that others will think, big deal, but for me and him they were massive:

- A good deal more canoodling.
- Being able to book a Lake District cottage for Christmas instead of stocking up on drink.
- Losing weight (now size 12 from a 16!)
- Writing again, and I count these blogs as getting motivated to do it, and settling enough to read more.
- Saying no to people who make me sad or intimidate me.
- Thinking about how to develop this new self-awareness further so I can help others in some way.

To anyone who already knows how wonderful it is to have the positive experience of AF, thank you for pushing me and helping me along, To those who are still confused about what part of AF is actually beneficial in their lives, PLEASE consider the positives and take a hold of all the wonderful possibilities out there for you when you are FREE.

I sensed my continuous daily blogging phase was slowing to every few days, not because I was fed up, but because daily blogging had done its job for me. I loved reading other people's and was so thrilled to hear good news, and so pleased to be able to help a little if people were feeling bad. But this desperate urge to get it all down was lessening. I decided that this meant that I'd expunged a lot of the things that were stopping me getting better. I thought this looking around me and deciding to move on a bit was a healthy thing. I am overjoyed to be one of the non-drinkers who are binning off the Drink Demon FOR EVER because they say:

1. I want to keep my liver, kidneys, bladder, stomach, bowels, throat, and breasts free of cancer for as long as

possible.

2. I don't want to have a stroke because I've drunk and smoked too much,

3. I don't want to be in the same boat as people who act like arseholes in town and upset everyone.

4. I want more money in my purse/wallet for important stuff, like spending quality time with my husband.

5. I want to have self-esteem.

6. I want to be respected for not drinking.

7. I want people to confide in me and for me to be able to help them with a clear head.

8. I want to get up in the morning and look forward to the day with no hangover.

9. I want my husband to be proud of me and trust me.

10. I want to fulfil my dreams.

11. I want to think of my bucket list and know I have a fighting chance of doing the things on it.

12. I want to help my new AF friends stay AF.

13. I want to feel feelings and think thoughts.

14. I want to be able to distinguish between feelings and facts with clarity.

15. I want to lose weight healthily and have the motivation to be genuinely fit and healthy.

16. I want money for hobbies and interests like my garden and eventually, one day, getting back on a horse.

17. I want to go on holiday in future and not spend most of it feeling hungover.

18. I want to stop arguing and the arguments going sky high.

19. I want my PMS to ease off and stay eased off.

20. I want my face to still look fresh in ten, or even twenty years' time.

21. I don't want people to pity me.

22. I want to lead, not be lead.

23. I want to be a role model.

24. I want to value my achievements.

25. I want to help others have achievements they value.

26. I want a fit, sexy body.

27. I want my hair to be sleek and long and shiny.

28. I don't want to be malnourished any more.

29. I want to go on holiday without obsessing where the alcohol will be.

30. I want to have even moods and be known as an even person.

31. I want enough time freed up to do new stuff, or get better at the stuff I already do.

32. I want to have the energy to be creative.

33. I want to sleep properly.

34. I don't want to hate myself.

35. I don't want to keep funding supermarkets any more than I absolutely have to.

36. I want to use less glass, packaging, and other environmentally damaging rubbish associated with drinking.

37. I don't want to be dumbed down.

38. I want to understand my personality and motivations.

39. I want to like myself.

40. I don't want to be thought of as weak, moody, or ineffectual at work because I am always ill or down.

41. I don't want to be a drug addict.

42. I don't want to feel thirsty all the time.

43. I want a different routine.

44. I want the second half of my life to be productive and worthwhile.

45. I don't want to look back at bad memories any more, or create any more.

46. I don't want to feel sorry for myself and expect others to solve all my problems – I want to take responsibility.

47. I don't want to lie to myself or be in denial.

48. I want to be in control.

49. I don't want to feel so worried and anxious that I cannot function normally.

50. I don't want to tell any more lies.

51. I don't to have any more awful secrets.

52. I want space to forgive myself and others.

53. I want to feel confident about being unique.

54. I want to inspire others to action.

55. I don't want to be afraid.

56. I want to continue to feel liberated from prison.

57. I want to come and go as I please without organising life round a drink.

58. I want to be independent minded.

59. I want to laugh at life.

60. I want to plan my future with confidence.

61. I want to lay down roots.

62. I want to make commitments I stick to.

63. I want to be proactive.

64. I want to stop taking medication to get through the day.

65. I don't want a crutch.

66. I want to be discerning.

67. I want to be in tune with my body and respect it.

68. I want to know everything will be all right.

69. I want to enjoy long walks and cycles without a crippling headache, and have the energy to make full use of outside leisure time without craving my bed.

70. I want to stop wasting time.

71. I want to stop others wobbling or blipping or denying.

72. I want to make plans I can stick to.

73. I want to stop people pleasing.

74. I want to say no (or yes if the situation requires it) with confidence.

75. I want to take calculated rather than crazy risks.

76. I want to have genuine not drug-induced fun.

77. I want to feel like a girl again.

78. I want to remember what made me feel good when I was young.

79. I want to set my own boundaries.

80. I don't want to hide.

81. I want to study for new qualifications and not score mediocre marks because my head is banging.

83. I want to help others by writing and do so without having a glass by my side.

84. I don't want to be a hypocrite guiding and advising people in my job when I am a mess at home.

85. I want to be a revolutionary.

86. I want to do things my way.

87. I want to have enough head space to consider my actions before I make too hasty decisions.

88. I want to be a coach, to myself and others.

89. I want to like life.

90. I want to want to get old.

91. I don't want to hear rattling bottles in my shopping bag anymore.

92. I want to run a 10k in a good time and not sink a bottle of red as soon as I get in as some kind of reward.

93. I never want alcohol as a present ever again.

94. I want healthy, unbitten nails.

95. I want to keep my temper.

96. I don't want to catastrophise any more.

97. I want to believe that there are not problems, only challenges.

98. I want to allow people to tell me truths and not get upset with them.

99. I want to be able to tell others truths and not get upset doing it.

100. I want to achieve all of the above.

Other titles by Accent Press

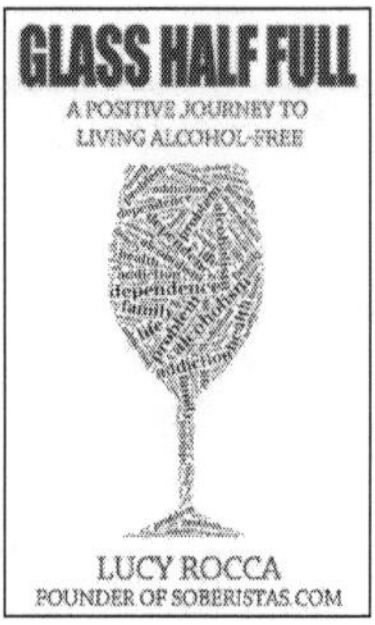

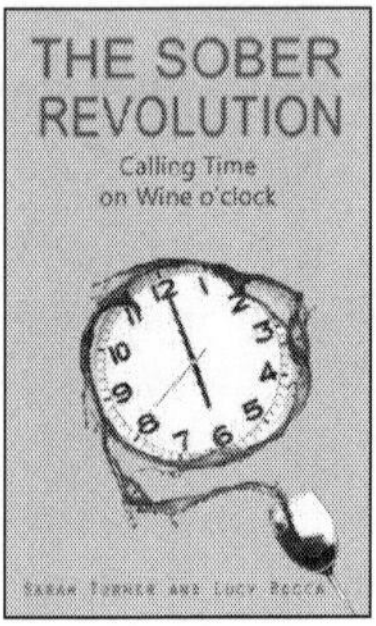

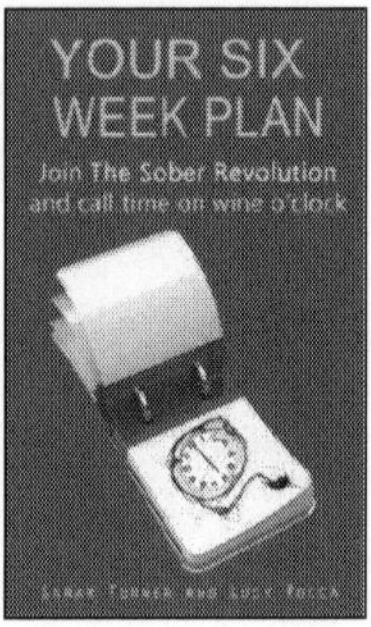

For more information about Binki Laidler

and other Accent Press titles

please visit

www.accentpress.co.uk

6838736R00124

Printed in Great Britain
by Amazon.co.uk, Ltd.,
Marston Gate.